Between Two Worlds

ELLEN P. YOUNG

Between Two Worlds

Special Moments
of Alzheimer's & Dementia

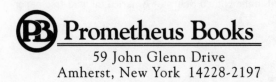 **Prometheus Books**

59 John Glenn Drive
Amherst, New York 14228-2197

Published 1999 by Prometheus Books

Inquiries should be addressed to
Prometheus Books, 59 John Glenn Drive, Amherst, New York 14228–2197.
VOICE: 716–691–0133, ext. 207. FAX: 716–564–2711.
WWW.PROMETHEUSBOOKS.COM

03 02 01 00 99   5 4 3 2 1

Library of Congress Cataloging-in-Publication Data

Young, Ellen P.
    Between two worlds : special moments of Alzheimer's & dementia / Ellen P. Young.
        p.   cm.
    Includes bibliographical references.
    ISBN 1–57392–697–3 (alk. paper)
    1. Alzheimer's disease Anecdotes. 2. Dementia Anecdotes. I. Title.
RC523.2.Y68   1999
362.1'96831—dc21   99–14643
                                                                         CIP

Printed in the United States of America on acid-free paper

For my beloved mother,
who throughout her life has had a
never-ending sense of whimsy,
and for her beautiful sister
who had a special grace and positive attitude until the end.

Contents

Acknowledgments

The secret to bringing this book alive was being fortunate enough to have people open their hearts and share their stories with me. It was an amazing experience to encounter such courage in the face of such adversity. My heartfelt thanks to all those wonderful people who cared enough about others to partake in this project. It is hoped that the book will not only provide stories with which to identify, but also provide support for anyone involved in dealing with dementia at any level. It is also hoped that the book will do well in order that the royalties may make a substantial contribution to the Alzheimer's Association toward research for a cure.

Very special thanks go to the Central Maryland Chapter of the Alzheimer's Association in Baltimore. Its executive director, Cass Naugle, really paved my way. The contributions made by Edna Ellett, Tom and Dolly Wheatley, Evelyn McLay, Don South, and Maureen Pullias were invaluable.

Thanks also to the friends, co-workers, and physicians who

were supportive of this venture and contributed material to it. I appreciate all the support from Peter Rabins, M.D., Allen Genut, M.D., and Michael Gloth, M.D. Terry Jacobus, Carol Gamble, Lynn Rosenberg, Anne Keene, and June Cole also deserve special mention as do Gloria Jean Hammel, Lynn Shuppel, Mary Riley, Jean Tucker Mann, Sister Genevieve Kunkel, SSND, and Judy Joyce. This book would never have gone to press without Steven L. Mitchell, Cindy Seide, Hirsh Goldberg, and David Pessin.

Finally, and personally most important, my heart is full of gratitude and love for my children, Wayne Verity, Lynne Verity Flynn, and her husband, Michael Flynn, who provided me with immeasurable love and support through it all.

Foreword

by Peter V. Rabins, M.D., MPH

Alzheimer disease has worked its way into public consciousness and is now recognized as a common illness with serious public health consequences. What is most intriguing is that it is not a new disease, like AIDS, but rather has been known to affect humankind for 10,000 years—as long as there has been the written word.

How, then, can we understand the fact that Alzheimer disease was unknown thirty years ago? The answer partly relates to the increasing number of individuals living into old age and the resultant increase in the number of people at risk of developing Alzheimer disease. More importantly, however, is the recognition by the scientific and medical communities that what was once dismissed as "just senility" is a specific disease that was described in the beginning of the twentieth century by Dr. Alois Alzheimer.

Why, if Dr. Alzheimer described the disease at the turn of the century, was Alzheimer disease not recognized as the most common cause of cognitive decline in the elderly until the late 1960s? Clearly, the answer is that medical and scientific communities had ignored dementia and Alzheimer disease and had not done the careful research needed to understand the causes of "senility" until then.

A third element that has contributed greatly to our appreciation of the need for better care for those suffering from Alzheimer disease has been the demands placed by family members on society to provide better services, more understanding, and more knowledge.

Between Two Worlds is a wonderful example of the benefits that can come from focusing attention on an illness. By helping us understand what the person with the disease goes through and what that person's loved ones experience, this book helps humanize what is a sad and heroic struggle against the ravages of a difficult disease. By showing us that a sense of humor is as important as an appreciation of the disease's devastation, *Between Two Worlds* provides an important lesson addressing the devastation of this illness and the positives that can result. For while the pain experienced by the patient and family needs to be appreciated, the ability of human beings to respond to difficult circumstances is extraordinary. By showing both the pain and the positive, *Between Two Worlds* demonstrates that difficult problems can be overcome by facing them head on and appreciating the bad and the good that they bring.

Peter V. Rabins, M.D., MPH
Professor of Psychiatry
Johns Hopkins University School of Medicine
Baltimore, Maryland

Foreword

by Allan Genut, M.D.

Wouldn't it be nice for children to be born with graduate degrees already in hand, or at least able to communicate? How about being born with just basic social graces—like toilet training? We cherish young children and newborns though they start with no senses of their own. They must be exposed to light to develop sight, sound to develop hearing, and touch to thrive. Shortly these and other senses are blended, as if by magic, in the process of learning, communication, and creativity—processes that will continue for a lifetime.

A patient with dementia, unfortunately, goes in reverse; losing first creativity, then ability to learn, then communication, and eventually even perception. Though there is little difference cognitively between an infant and a demented patient, the joy of the former is in soaring upward and the desolation of the latter is in the regression downward.

I chose to be a neurologist, knowing full well that some of my patients would have devastating and incurable disorders. My meager role with these patients is to help them get through it in the best possible way. Of all incurable patients, I have the least to offer to those with Alzheimer's disease. That's why I read with awe and admiration about Ellen Young's journey with these patients and their caregivers. Despite their unraveling cognition, she found the wondrous child in each of them. In so doing, she impaled the monster that is Alzheimer's right through the heart.

But it is as much her literary talent as her positive thinking that makes this work such a gem. Vignettes, short or long, are woven into an epic tale of courage and human dignity in the face of the greatest of all adversities. The message is the heroism that is inherent in all humanity, caregiver and receiver alike.

Ellen's book is not only for those who have been touched by Alzheimer's disease, but contains much that is of interest to all of us. Though most of us would not, of our own free will, choose to be entertained by a work on Alzheimer's disease, this is truly a book that, once started, cannot be put down.

Allan Genut, M.D.
Neurologist
Baltimore, Maryland

Preface

You grow up the day you have your first real laugh at yourself.
—Ethel Barrymore

Alzheimer's, AIDS, cancer—all strike terror in our hearts when we hear the diagnosis. Until the much-needed medical break-throughs come along and cures or vaccines are found, we have to find ways to deal with our fears. I am hoping that this book will help serve as a kind of "fear buster." By staring the Alzheimer's monster down and even laughing a little in the face of it, we bolster our courage and literally release the kind of chemicals in ourselves that help us to gain more of a sense of well-being in the face of adversity.

Alzheimer's disease is a progressive neurological disorder of middle and old age characterized by impairment first in one, then another, and finally, all areas of cognition. Memory is most often affected first, but abstract thought, self-awareness, language, judgment, and attention are also often lost early. Later, inability to perform the activities of daily living, confusion, incontinence, disturbances of behavior and emotional response, and psychosis occur in many patients. Even motor skills can sometimes become severely impaired.

In the terminal phase, some patients become vegetative while others have no awareness of the world around them.

Early in the disease process, the more stimulation the brain receives, the slower the deterioration. In recent years the University of Kentucky has conducted a "Nuns' Study." Studies of orders of nuns who are highly educated and receive constant mental stimulation indicate a dramatically lower incidence of Alzheimer's. Thus far there is no cure. There are very few medical interventions, but a lot is happening in research and a breakthrough may be near. One of the main purposes for writing this book is to raise funds for research for a cure.

A family struck by Alzheimer's is a family in crisis. A family is a unit (though sometimes scattered), and the "whole family" must be considered, in terms of caregiving. Although there is often one designated caregiver, other family members can offer respite care, emotional support, and possibly financial support. With good communication, they can function as a "whole." Although that may seem like the best of all possible worlds, it is truly what is best for the patient and for the family.

Much has been written about how to make caregiving easier and more efficient. Caregivers have been advised to consider their own health and take a break when necessary. Little has been written about considering humor as a tool with which to make life easier for both the patient and the caregiver. I hope to make this work a forum for that humor.

It is my belief that a silver lining can be found in most situations, if we look hard enough. It's not just a Pollyanna attitude. It's a reality. This does not negate the fact, however, that there are some clouds that are not redeemed by silver linings, however bright.

So, this is a book about love and pain, a book about taking a peek behind that darkest cloud and finding that gentle humor is often our greatest ally.

Even if no one you know has Alzheimer's, the disease still has a great impact on your life. There are now 4 million Americans with Alzheimer's. The total cost of caring for them is $50 billion in direct cost and $90 billion if indirect costs are included. If no cure is found, the number of cases will swell to 14 million by 2020 and 40 million by 2050, with a total care cost of $1 trillion per year. Even the most affluent country on Earth could not pay that bill.

—Allan Genut, M.D.

Introduction

As we approach a new millennium, there seems to be a global spiritual hunger that is becoming more and more evident. Many are still satisfied with their own religious mainstream traditions, but many others are seeking new ways to try to understand and accept the universe as it unfolds. Books on near-death experiences, New Age philosophy, and love stories depicting great sacrifice are just a few of the present-day phenomena.

Alzheimer's disease itself has nothing spiritual about it. But the effect of the disease process on all those surrounding the afflicted one can either be devastating or can provide a challenge. Having already lost an aunt to Alzheimer's, things are moving inexorably toward the second loss—my mother. My career is in social work. I am based in a hospital as a medical social worker, where a substantial portion of my cases have involved Alzheimer's patients and their families. I have been doing discharge planning and counseling for fifteen years. Discharge planning involves making the necessary arrangements for patients when they leave the hospital, i.e., nursing home placement or assisted living arrangements. Experience prior to that includes a children's institutional setting, working with the elderly in the community, and every conceivable family problem from marital counseling to addictions.

I believe we need to galvanize our spiritual energies to help ourselves overcome, or at least better cope with, the fear, as well as the mental and physical exhaustion generated in families who are dealing with Alzheimer's disease. The writing of this book has been a kind of catharsis for me. It has helped me to work through some of my own grief and feelings of helplessness in the face of the ravages caused by this disease to my loved ones. It has also helped me see through some of the painful moments to the other side, where mirth can sometimes be accessed. Plainly speaking, it has helped me to laugh, sometimes in spite of myself, at some of the endlessly repetitive questions and antics that come from the "dementia-challenged" person.

The material in this book is positive and humorous while respectful of the individual struggles of Alzheimer's patients and their families. The primary aim is to lighten the load and lessen the burden felt by anyone who has ever been, is currently, or ever will be involved with Alzheimer's disease, at any level. This envelops the patients, families, caregivers, and those working with Alzheimer's in any capacity.

People who are still in the very sensitive early stages of dealing with a loved one who is suffering from Alzheimer's or a related dementia may have some difficulty with the concept of "accessing mirth" in the patient/caregiver relationship. Those who will benefit most from this book are people who, at times, are able to laugh at their own expense. For example, when I can't find my keys, I continue to remind myself that it isn't "not finding the keys" that's a problem. It is not knowing what to do with them when they are found that would be a legitimate, all kidding aside, warning sign of trouble on the frontier.

I recently saw a program that featured physically challenged comedians whose routine was primarily jokes about their own situations. They were amputees and partially paralyzed men and women, most of whom had been in some kind of terrible accident. Each one of them said that humor was what got them through the pain, the frustration, the anger, the depression, and the confusion in their altered lives. The phrase "access mirth," that I have coined and will use throughout this book, describes what those comedians were doing. The extraordinary part of their stage routines was that the comic material made use of their own efforts to live with their handicaps and some of the ordeals they faced in that attempt. Another related phenomenon was described on a documentary series called *The Human Animal* that was hosted by Phil Donahue and aired many years ago. Clowns and comedians are shown going into a hospital to visit patients who are in severe pain, some of whom are in traction. The point is to show that laughter releases endorphins (the happy brain chemicals), that in turn, do as good a job, if not better, than painkillers. This is not some hokey idea, it is a fact. Take note, the next time you have a good laugh, of the feeling of well-being that comes over you.

My hope is that together, caregivers, family members, and even patients can turn things around a little bit, change some of our perceptions, and access a different view of the daily trials and tribulations of dealing with dementia. This includes dementia of any type, Alzheimer's related, stroke related, or the many reversible dementias that come from kidney failure, diabetic reactions, chemical imbalances in the brain, or toxic reactions to drugs. Whatever the cause, the family or friends of people so afflicted have to deal with the results, be it on a temporary or permanent basis. The closer one is to the problem, the harder it is to be objective or to have a philosophical viewpoint. It is definitely a challenge to focus on some of the real humor that is part of many of the behaviors of the average Alzheimer's patient. There are some patients, however, who have nothing about them that could be interpreted as humorous. It is hoped that their numbers are relatively few, but for those who care for them, it is important to remember that the loved one is probably not suffering physical pain and may be unaware of any other kind of discomfort. Caregivers can't be caregivers for others unless they take care of themselves.

For the caregivers who are able to "access mirth" either during or after their ordeal, this book provides a forum for their strength, a monument to their courage, and a chance to relive those humorous memories that will keep their loved ones close to them for many years to come.

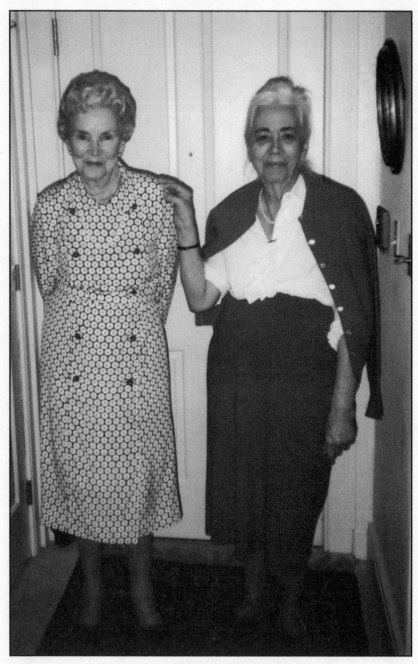

Mother (at right) and Auntie Peg

Chapter 1

"Please Don't Eat the Marigold"

It was two seconds, literally, to Auntie Peg's room from my office as a social worker in the hospital. I planned a quick stop around lunchtime as I had been checking on her throughout the morning. A companion (aide) was with her, and as I entered the room I heard, "Oh Sweetheart, please don't eat the marigold. That's just to make your tray look pretty!" Auntie Peg smiled her usual beatific smile and put down the remains of the blossom. As the companion began feeding her, she looked over at me. I took note of the mirth dancing around the corners of her eyes and mouth; discreetly, of course, in respect for Auntie Peg's dignity, as she was still a very dignified woman. All eighty-five years of her life, she had literally defined the word.

This brief anecdote is just one of many that I experienced during the period I spent as caregiver of my aunt. Although she lived in the healthcare center of a retirement facility and the nurses and aides met all her basic care needs, I was the overseer of things in general. "Things in general" can get to be quite involved when you have a mother who is showing signs of traveling down the same path and you are also her caregiver. Mother had recently entered a nearby nursing home and was making a relatively good adjustment. Leaving her apartment willingly, but not happily, for what seemed to her like the final stop, was not easy.

Not long after the marigold incident, my aunt became an angel. She died right in my arms. My daughter and I knew that she was immediately in the celestial realm because the movie *Sister Act* was playing on the other patient's TV and the nuns were singing Gregorian Chant. After all, what other proof would we need? This had to be more than a coincidence!

Now it may, at "first thought," appear to some that mirth and death don't go together. Birth and death are connected, that we know, but mirth, humor, a chuckle or two around issues like death and sometimes worse yet, Alzheimer's—oh no, can't be!

Alzheimer's causes "dis-ease" for the patient and all loved ones. Dis-ease is something that compromises or removes completely our sense of well-being, our "ease." It is sometimes a toss-up as to who suffers more, the patient or the caregiver. There are various times and stages at which patients can be aware of what is happening to them. For caregivers, however, especially those living with the patient, every day truly does become a "36-hour day." There is endless daily repetition and tedium that can tear at a person's very soul. The level of dis-ease for the caregiver can sometimes reach the point of breakdown and inability to continue. I see this frequently in the hospital where I do medical social work. Tired, frustrated, confused, and sometimes angry and resentful, caregivers often confront their day with sagging shoulders, darkened eye sockets, obvious weight loss or gain, a sense of helplessness and hopelessness. Beyond what my clinical knowledge can provide, having been there myself helps me to understand what they are going through.

"Laughter is the best medicine." Just an old saying, or is there some truth there? It is a good form of free self-medication according to those who have written about the therapeutic effects of endorphin-releasing giggles. Books like *Laughing Your Way to Good Health* by Susan Vass and all the Norman Cousins contributions are good examples of this phenomenon. Now comes the big question. What can we possibly find to laugh about when someone has the grave misfortune of being diagnosed (conditionally, as positive diagnosis can only be made from a postmortem of the brain tissue) with Alzheimer's disease? Laughter about anything related to this tragedy could seem rather cavalier, irreverent, or even insolent. People can be very sensitive about their illnesses. When something is serious, it's serious, and do we really want to laugh at times like these?

I propose to you that we do. I further propose to you that if we do not inject some mirth into these perfectly dreadful situations, our hearts and souls will die more than just a little, right along with our loved ones. The word love as in "loved ones" gives us a clue. Love is gentle, love is kind, love is forgiving. These are the words that are frequently linked with love. Another word frequently linked with love in the self-help world is "tough." "When the going gets tough, the tough get going." There are many well-known sayings about love, but saying and doing are far apart. I propose that the caregivers of Alzheimer's and related dementia patients get tough in the most loving possible way.

First, we look at the family system. If it is only you and the patient, look at that relationship. Then we ask ourselves, honestly, the following questions. What would we want if the positions were reversed and we were the dementia victim? Is everyone in the family system being considered equally or have we targeted the patient to be front and center in all ways, to the possible exclusion of our own emotional and physical well-being? If a case is made for the fact that we have put ourselves in the background then we must be called to attention here. We should start to pay some attention to ourselves and other loved ones besides the patient. Perhaps many of us are getting a bit frayed around the edges.

For those fortunate enough to have strong faith, it could be said that faith will sustain them. It will, for those who have it, if they remember the master commandment—"do unto others. . . ." Treat others the way you would want them to treat you and try to care for them the way you care for yourself. We already started to address what we would want if we traded places with the patient. No doubt most of us would not want to tax our children or relatives beyond their limits and we would be frequently telling them that they should take care of themselves. Caring about your neighbor as you care about yourself is often misunderstood. When the statement is examined closely, one realizes it implies that first you must care about yourself, and then try to care about others the same way. If we drop in our tracks from exhaustion and self-neglect, who are we helping? After all, we're all in it together, like it or not. These may be tricky or difficult concepts but they are offered, nevertheless, as food for thought.

A very brave woman by the name of Diana Friel McGowin, an early-onset Alzheimer's victim, wrote her own story titled *Living in the Labyrinth*. (Presenile or early-onset Alzheimer's-type dementia begins before age sixty-five). McGowin says, "It is essential that the patient and family try their utmost to keep a healthy sense of humor alive. There are some opprobrious situations which will befall you and your only salvation will be the grace of laughter. It provides the same venting release as a scream, but is much more socially acceptable." This lady had an IQ of 137 and a vocabulary that just wouldn't quit. It had me running to the dictionary more than once.

So let's get to work and release some endorphins. Remember those happy little chemicals in the brain? Laughter and chocolate are two things that make the happy juices flow! A friend, Pat, told me a story about her father who suffered from dementia brought on by a stroke not long before he died. The family had finally persuaded him to give up the car keys and give the car to his son-in-law. The following Sunday when the family started out for church, Dad looked out the window and said, "Where's my car?"

"You gave it to Ray last week, don't you remember?"

Dad looked puzzled for a minute and then said indignantly, "That was a damn dumb thing to do. Now I'll have to go out and buy a new one!" Dad was quite a character. Can't you just see that whole scenario as it unfolded?

Another family member told me that his mother calls him from her nursing home room and the conversation goes something like this:

"Hello, Bruce, how are you?"

"Okay, Mom, how are you doing?"

"Bruce, where are you—and—and where am I? I don't know this place."

Bruce proceeds to tell his mother where he lives and then tells her the name of the nursing home and how long she has been there.

"Bruce, you must have gone crazy—I've never been in this place before in my life!"

Bruce says his mother had always been a very nervous, anxious person. Since she has suffered from what has been diagnosed as having Alzheimer's-type dementia, she has seemed more content. It appears she can't recall what she used to worry about so she just enjoys the moment. (Incidentally, she is still able to dial Bruce's number on the telephone when she's having a good day.) She does well in the dementia program where she spends two hours a day. The rest of the time she is in her room with the TV as a companion. As any professional caregiver will tell you, interaction with people is better for Alzheimer's patients because it stimulates them. But TV can make a fairly stimulating companion for some dementia patients. Even if their concentration is impaired to the point of not being able to follow the story line, they can still respond to the happenings of the moment, particularly humor. My mother laughs whenever we watch the video of Victor Borge and his piano antics. Having played the piano herself, she always comments that she wishes he'd play more and horse around less.

Faith, support, and mirth play an important role in getting us through. The reason I feel qualified to be on a soapbox about this topic is that I have walked the walk. Those good at talking the talk from working with others or from a clinical model are much appreciated, but there is nothing that teaches with as much certainty as experience itself. Experience informs us about ourselves. It brings to light things that hitherto may have been unknown to us. It teaches us about the depth of our capacities to be patient, kind, forbearing, and most of all, unconditionally loving. For unconditional love is the best we can give our Alzheimer's loved ones. Early-stage patients tell us how much they long to know they will be lovingly and patiently cared for. Their capacity for understanding any negative behavior toward them dwindles rapidly and they become easily frightened and dejected.

There is an old adage, corny as it may sound: Laugh and the world laughs with you, cry and you cry alone. People avoid pity-party types. They gravitate toward those who try to be positive even in the face of adversity. Caregivers can easily fall into the self-pity trap because they truly *do* carry a burden and the only thing that is going to relieve them is death itself. Thinking too much about that or wishing too much for it to happen brings on feelings of guilt, though there are certainly times when even those kinds of thoughts are appropriate. For example, if a loved one is suffering a great deal.

One caregiver, who we will call Judy, told me she had to do battle with her siblings when she told them of their mother's diagnosis.

"Are you trying to tell me our mother is a nut case!?" her brother snapped.

The mother went downhill very fast and actually became nonverbal with the exception of moments of lucidity that were like bright flashes when she would say something appropriate. One day as Judy helped her mother into a pink flowered dress, her mother looked very serious and said loudly, "Gauche!" She hadn't spoken in months!

"You know, mother, you're a real comedian," chuckled Judy. Her mother hesitated a moment, then joined in the laughter. She could still walk reasonably well and suddenly turned on her heels and walked down the hall, swearing loudly as she went. One of the last truly patrician ladies swearing away! Is there anything else to do but laugh? You could try crying but I'll bet it wouldn't help as much.

Did you know that the chemicals found in tears of sadness and tears of laughter are different? Both provide relief and generally make us feel better, but tears produced by laughter generate a real high. It follows that if we feel better we radiate more positive vibes and everyone around us feels better as a result, including our loved ones afflicted with Alzheimer's.

Remember the man who gave his car to his son-in-law and then wondered what he had done with it? He must have missed his true calling as a comedian. Another car incident occurred when he was at his daughter Pat's house for a family gathering. Someone had driven his car there and parked it in the driveway. It seemed to calm him down if he could see his car. He wasn't as likely to nag about wanting to drive. This particular day, however, that strategy didn't work. He became agitated and insisted that he wanted to drive himself home. He was sure he knew the way. When no one tried to stop him, he got up, started to walk around the room, and said, "How the hell do you get out of here?" Much later, when he was completely bedridden and near death, he was being given a bed bath. At one point, he fairly rose up and shouted, "Stop trying to kill me, don't you know I'm a dying man?!" Earlier in his illness Pat reports that he kept thinking he was on a ship, probably due to the sense of imbalance that dementia patients sometimes experience. He kept saying, "When are they going to let us off this ship? I want to see Hawaii."

From a personal standpoint it took me many years to be able to think in anything but the most negative terms about Alzheimer's. Alzheimer's or cancer—how terrifying to imagine being diagnosed with either of those dreadful life intruders. Ironically, we sometimes hear stories about people who actually say they think of their disease as a gift. Even people with AIDS have been known to say that. Though it may sound a bit overdramatic, the people who feel this way may be those who didn't know how to really live their lives. Maybe they needed life to hit them over the head in order to learn to savor the moment and take time to smell the proverbial roses.

C. S. Lewis was an English novelist and essayist on theological and moral problems. Lewis says, "Pain is God's megaphone to rouse a deaf world." That is strong-sounding stuff. As thinking human beings we struggle constantly to make sense of a world that continually challenges our endurance of emotional and physical pain. There seems to be nowhere to legitimately place the anger we feel when something as critically important as pain and suffering is out of our control. We could philosophize and question forever, but we will never really understand suffering, even if we look at it under the microscope of all the world religions and great philosophies put together.

Is it comprehending the reasons for suffering or is it the ability to be flexible enough to accept it that is at issue here? What we can't understand, we either learn to somehow grudgingly accept or we choose to fight it with every bit of our energy, physically and emotionally. Our basic human instinct, when faced with danger, is fight or flight. The fight in this case depletes us of our needed energy, for our Alzheimer's loved ones and ourselves. Running away from anything burns up energy. In this case why not take flight, but in a uniquely metaphorical way; flight into mirth, flight into hope. Not in a neurotic, escapist way, but rather, flight into the reality of the situation. Stare the monster down. Take a good, long, painful look at what you're dealing with and then take yourself by the proverbial scruff of the neck, batten down the hatches, and say, "Let's get on with life while life is here to get on with." I tried exactly that and it worked!

Postscript

It has been five years since fingers first touched word processor to bring this book to life. The one constant in life is change, and needless to say, there has been some. The postscripts at the end of some of the chapters will serve as updates.

Starting with my own dear mother, there has been change. Incredibly, she is coming up to her eighty-ninth birthday. She no longer is mobile in any way, even with a walker. Weighing only one hundred pounds, she is moved from bed to a specially padded wheelchair and back, as needed. Still alert, she continues to be gracious and loving toward people, though communication has become more difficult. Much of what she says is garbled, but now and then something comes out clearly. She can still say "I love you."

Sometimes it seems almost as if Mother's whole life has been forgotten—everything except the present moment. She certainly has forgotten that there is something called death. She seems to have no intention of going anywhere at the moment.

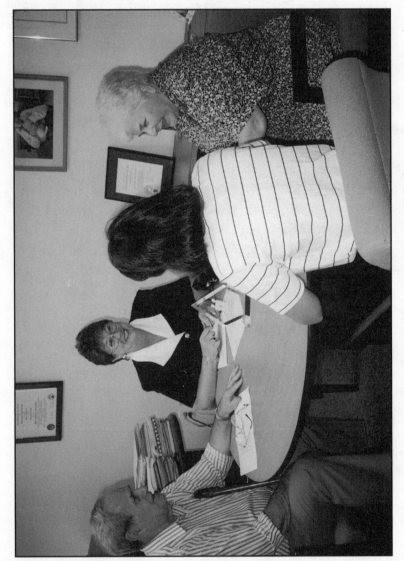

From left: Richard, Jean, Mary, and Martha

2

Support Group I

"Lost Between Two Worlds"

When I began working on this project, I visited the Central Maryland Chapter of the Alzheimer's Association here in Baltimore to attend a lunchtime meeting with several caregivers who were kind enough to share their stories with me, highlighting some of the humor. I will present four valuable scenarios that emerged from the meeting. My hope is to have caregivers who are reading this book, and are shut in at home, be able to feel as if they are actually part of a support group when they read this chapter and chapter 5, "Support Group II." It is sincerely hoped that they will be able to closely identify with the caregivers in these chapters.

For the sake of anonymity, I have given the caregivers fictitious names. Richard is a man who lost his wife to early-onset Alzheimer's. Martha's story is about her mother who lives with Martha and her husband. Jean's contribution is about her mother-in-law who lives with Jean and her husband. Mary presents the story of the single woman, who, unable to meet the care needs of her mother, must place her in a nursing home.

This chapter is as close to our original conversations as possible.

Richard: My wife, Jane, was an early-onset victim. She was only about forty-six when she first showed symptoms of dementia. We had been married about twenty years, had two daughters, twelve and thirteen. When the children were small I became disabled with multiple sclerosis and Jane took care of me. One of the most troublesome things that I had to cope with was the reaction of my two daughters. People look at things in life in different ways and my daughters did not cope with their mother's deterioration the same way that I did. It almost destroyed one of them. My elder daughter was a big help. In fact, I couldn't have done it without her.

One of the first strange things I noticed in Jane's behavior was that she kept writing "ice cream" on the shopping list over and over again. And she didn't even like ice cream! Even though she wrote it on the list over and over, nine times out of ten, she wouldn't bring it home.

When we were out for dinner and I'd ask her to tell me what she wanted, she would say, "Oh, whatever you're having is fine with me." It was the same with dessert. Then she wouldn't say a word; she'd just eat it.

One time we were in a doctor's office, sitting in the waiting room when a nurse came out and asked for Jane's age. She piped up, "None of your damn business." I almost passed out from the shock! I was really mad. There were a lot of people sitting there, and the nurse really shouldn't have asked in front of everybody. But the thing was, Jane had never minded talking about her age, so her reaction was a real jolt to me. When I asked her later why she had acted that way, she had no idea what I was talking about. She seemed completely indifferent. At the time, I just thought this was a reflection of the mood she was in. She could be very direct. During our life together, I had come up with some crazy ideas from time to time and when she said "No," it meant, "Forget it."

Things progressed, and one of the first incidents that gave me a big clue that something was very wrong happened one night when we had four friends over for dinner. I thought I'd make the dinner, we'd have a little party, and have a good time. At this point, I needed a diversion. After everyone arrived, my wife was walking around, seeming lost. At one point, someone was in the kitchen and called out to me that the microwave door was open. I left it that way when we were in the house alone, because it served as a mirror. There was also a mirror in the dining room and when I sat in the living room I could see her reflected from every angle. There was only one little space left uncovered, and if she stayed there too long, I'd get up to see what she was doing. Of course, that evening I just closed the door.

Back to the dinner party. We were sitting and having a couple of cocktails and one of the guests said to me, "By the way, didn't you invite us for dinner?" I answered in the affirmative and she said, "Well, Jane just cleaned up the kitchen. She put all the food down the garbage disposal." Well! What do you do? I mean, do you yell and scream or just make the best of it? We went out for pizza!

It soon got to the point that I had to have everything done ahead of time. Everything had to be hidden. Things were inside the oven or refrigerator, places she wouldn't be apt to look. We couldn't have any food out at all or she would put it right down the garbage disposal. Needless to say, this was all very hard on my daughters.

Jane was an avid reader and was always in the library. She read everything from what I call "mattress to mattress novels" to things in Old English. She just liked to read. She was very bright. Years later, at the nursing home, they would say, "But she's a schoolteacher—how could she have Alzheimer's?" I told them over and over again that that had nothing to do with it. As things got worse, though, when we'd go to the library, she wanted to take out all the books, but in the end she'd just be sitting there with the book upside down. She had been a fast reader. In fact when things started getting rough, she was still substitute teaching and her students just thought she was being a good sport when she would do "funny" things.

The principal contacted me and said, "Jane is always drinking."

"Drinking!?" I said.

"She is always leaving the classroom to go to the water fountain for a drink," he said.

I was perplexed by that because I knew she had been checked for diabetes, which can make you drink a lot, and didn't have it. In retrospect, though, it seemed to just be a stage. She would go through these phases and then it would pass. The way she could still pull herself together was amazing.

Shortly thereafter, things got really weird at school. Jane began to pull some tricks in the different schools where she would substitute. She killed all the goldfish in one school by feeding them dog biscuits! She said, "The dogs like them, why wouldn't the fish?" Finally, a letter was sent home to me. They called to tell me it was coming. They had already talked to her personally and were very concerned about her unpredictability. Her evaluation was poor because she was doing some crazy things. For instance, she loved animals and one day she let a dog that was in the playground into the school. That didn't go over so well. There were too many things going wrong, so I just pulled her out. Her teaching days were over.

By now I knew something was really wrong and I took her to a psychiatrist. He couldn't find any reason for her problems so I took her somewhere else. You see, in the beginning stages of Alzheimer's, people are like alcoholics. They can cover up a "multitude of sins," so to speak. If I asked Jane something and she couldn't figure out an answer, she would say, "Whatever you want is fine with me." There were lots of times when it wasn't so fine. Very soon, she was admitted to Johns Hopkins for a three-week evaluation. It was Eastertime. The doctors told me there was something wrong. They didn't think it was too serious, but they admitted they really didn't know. When she was home and several months had gone by, I called them to request another evaluation. Their response was, "But she was just here." She was going downhill fast; in fact, doing "power dives" at that point. Ultimately, they were amazed at how much she had deteriorated from April to August and they finally diagnosed it as Alzheimer's. (Many years later, when she died, the autopsy bore out the diagnosis.) At that point, when she was only in her early fifties, they thought she wouldn't last more than another year—maybe a year and a half.

So now, we were both at home. In the past, she had taken care of me and now it was my turn to take care of her. Looking back, in a strange way, it was somewhat satisfying to know we were living out our marital promises to each other. Life went on and our two daughters tried to keep things as normal as possible. Actually, it was better that I was at home or it would have been much harder on them. In the evening, after dinner, I'd do the dishes and Jane would watch TV. Ice-skating fascinated her. It calmed her down. The other things she'd watch were cartoons, especially *The Road-Runner*. (Later, it will be clear why that was certainly appropriate!) At one time, she loved opera and ballet but now she wouldn't watch either of them. I realized she couldn't follow the story line.

About six or seven years into the disease, before she was institutionalized, she was doing some strange things. Even more strange than usual. She said she was getting directions from someone else. It wasn't from me. One night we were in bed and I asked her if she had a friend, a secret friend. She looked at me as if she were thinking, "Should I tell him?" I'll never forget it. She then proceeded to tell me that it was a woman, a very nice person, who told her what to do. The woman had some friends, too. But I never saw her looking into the mirror or talking to anybody.

Then there was the toilet tissue incident. The rolls in the bathroom constantly disappeared. So when I came home from work or anyone visited, it was necessary to get out a new roll! I searched for them under the bed, in the closets—everywhere! Then one day, out of the blue, there they were—thirty-six rolls of toilet tissue on the bed. I had no idea where they came from. And that amount of toilet tissue is hard to hide! The fact that she remembered where she hid them was what amazed me. I then learned never to let on when I found a hiding place because she would keep using the same one. Once I found the mail in the couch but said nothing to her. From then on, I always knew where to look for it when it wasn't where it was supposed to be.

One time Jane took all my undershorts. Busy, busy, busy—she always had a project going. She hung them all on hangers, neatly, with earrings—using them as clips. Ironically, the earrings all matched!

Then came the point when I put her into adult day care, which was a lifesaver. When I'd pick her up from the program, she would start making faces at kids she saw in other cars. Of course they loved that and made faces right back. She'd stick her tongue out at them and I'd try to distract her by saying, "See what's in the glove compartment," and things like that. The kids would be looking, wanting more games, and there I was, trying to drive and distract her at the same time.

Early on, when I'd bring her home from the daycare center, she liked to take a walk around the block. She'd come home with a whole bunch of mail. She had taken the mail and newspapers from all the neighboring houses! The neighbors were understanding, and we returned the mail, but the newspapers were a little more difficult. It was hard to know to whom they belonged. Finally, one or two of the neighbors got a bit annoyed. I didn't blame them. People pay for their papers and they want to get them. Yeah—it was something. It was different, that's for sure.

There was a support group for caregivers at the daycare

center that was very helpful. One day a woman told a story about taking her husband out for the day. He was waiting for her to arrive and started talking to another visitor. He was trying to explain why he was there and what was wrong with him. He knew it began with A, but couldn't get Alzheimer's out. So instead he said, "I have AIDS."

During our thirty-two years of marriage, Jane's family and I never grew fond of one another. As the dementia progressed, Jane would tell them stories about me and when they would come to visit, they looked at me like I was some kind of "scuzz-ball"! I decided I'd call them on what I suspected they thought—that I was making a lot of Jane's problems up. So I sent her to visit them. They lived in another state, which necessitated a bus trip. They met her at the bus station. It was amazing how well she could hold it together for a short visit. So I called and asked if she could stay a little longer. They agreed and the next night she climbed out the window and went up the road, hitchhiking! She was found wandering around. Finally the family admitted that she was doing all the things I had been telling them about. I felt somewhat vindicated, as now they knew. Looking back, I think part of their problem was denial and their own fear of getting Alzheimer's.

Time went by. I had always thought I could put up with a lot. Like anything else in life, I felt I could tolerate five or even ten years of it. But when it went on and on, it only got harder. I kept Jane home until the last six years of the approximate full sixteen years of her illness. Of course, it had been coming on for a lot longer than I had realized. I had always said I wouldn't place her in a nursing home, but her doctor kept saying that's where she should be. She got to be so fast; she was like the *Road-Runner* cartoon. For example, every time we were in a doctor's office she'd go around and take everything off the walls before I could even stop her. There were times when she left the house without my knowing it. I'd think she was in the other room and she'd be out hitchhiking on a nearby highway. A call would come in saying someone had her someplace! After she had been in the nursing home for only three months, I told my elder daughter that I thought I could bring her home and try to manage again. My daughter said, "No way!"

One of the memories that stands out, in terms of events that could be considered humorous, was when it came time for her to go to the nursing home. She understood what was happening and began to pace constantly day and night, like an animal. It would drive me crazy. So I bought her a pair of comfortable shoes to at least save her feet. I gave her the shoes and she put them on and continued pacing. Then a little later she was in the bathroom and I heard this sloshing sound. I went to see what was going on and found her with one foot in the toilet. I was really frustrated and angry that she was ruining the new shoes. She looked at me and said nothing. But that look said a thousand words. A minute later she had the other foot in, just continuing to flush the toilet and watch the water run over the shoe. Now, that was a pivotal moment for me. The brand-new shoes were being ruined and I knew that I was either going to lose it completely or laugh. The expression on her face when she saw my distress was so comical. It clearly said, "You simple fool, can't you see that I'm making sure they're clean?!"

While we are on the topic of water sports, Jane was a great swimmer and was never afraid of water. Some Alzheimer's patients become frightened of water. The first time I tried to get her to take a shower instead of a bath, she just stood in the corner and looked at the water. By then she didn't know enough to put the soap to the washcloth. Instead, she just stood there looking at it. I tried to wash her from outside the shower but realized that it wasn't working when I started getting drenched. So I said, "Oh, what the hell," took my clothes off, and got right in with her. I found that was the only way to do it. Of course, my situation was entirely different from someone caring for a parent. Being married really helps in terms of bathing the patient!

When Jane was in the nursing home and really physically

deteriorating, my daughters had trouble with it—watching it happen, that is. My wife's brother wasn't able to handle it at all. He looked like he was ready to pass out when he saw her. The head nurse said, "You'll never see him again!" She had deteriorated so much. She didn't speak at all for the last three years. Trying to communicate with her was like talking to the wall.

The nursing home provided recreational therapy and sometimes they would bake cakes. One day my wife was coming toward me down the hall and I thought, "What's that in her mouth?" The nurse said, "It's an egg, a raw egg!" The egg was in the shell! We managed to get it out without breaking it. Then they used it in the cake! Anything and everything went in Jane's mouth. There's a lot about Alzheimer's that resembles early childhood. People who are severely demented can still recite the prayers of their childhood and bless themselves. Such embedded lessons last forever. Another resident had been a storekeeper. It was really quite amazing. Even when she literally no longer knew beans from bananas, she was still able to add and subtract perfectly. Another woman would sit in the hall all the time in a wheelchair. I noticed her there for about two years. She would just look at you and smile when you passed her. I thought she was mute. Well, one day when I was walking down the hall, holding my wife's hand, with her arm around me, this woman looked up and said real loudly, "There's a bed right down there— go to it!" She never said another word after that. Also, around the holidays, they had Santa Claus at the home and Jane found out he had candy. She wouldn't let him out of the place. She grabbed him going down the hall and tried to get more candy.

Once when I visited Jane in the nursing home, I found her face to be swollen. She had eaten some kind of a plant—they said they couldn't find which one. That was the only mistake made by the nursing home, though. In general, they were very good and took the group on a lot of outings. Once they took them to an aquarium. I thought they would be interested in the dol-

phins and the fish, but basically it bombed. There was a fish petting zoo upstairs, where you could actually handle the fish. The
director was showing my wife a starfish, when she grabbed it and
put it in her mouth. The fish blew up in size and became like
rubber. They weren't too happy. We had killed one of their
starfish! But that was the problem—beads, cigarette butts, anything, went right into her mouth.

One time at the nursing home, I just happened to say to Jane,
"You see these white hairs? You gave me every one of them."
She laughed and laughed. She thought that was the funniest thing
she had ever heard! Jane didn't speak for the last three years of
her life. She could speak. There was nothing physically wrong
that prevented her from speaking. She just forgot how. There was
a woman in the room with her who yelled and screamed all the
time. One day, out of the blue, my wife sat up and shouted, "Shut
up!" That was the last thing she ever said.

I knew she would die. We knew it was coming. They called at
5:00 A.M. and my first reaction was, "I'm free, it's over." That may
sound terrible. But then in about five minutes the realization set in
that she was no longer lost between two worlds. That was the only
way I could look at it. The expression in her eyes, the terror she
felt when things weren't going right, had been awful to watch. My
daughters were relieved and devastated at the same time.

(At this point, Richard, a brave and dedicated caregiver,
became a little teary. It had been three years since his wife died
but the wound was still visible. What an amazing story of love
and dedication. And what a testimony to the grace and strength
of the human spirit.)

Martha: My mother was extremely depressed after my father
died. She was a highly emotional person for most of her life,
always crying and feeling sorry for herself. Everybody else had it

better! You know, the classic pity-party-type person. She became very dependent on my brother and me. She really didn't care about other people, didn't have any friends. Only her immediate family counted all of her life. After my father died, she wanted friends, but it was too late then. I tried to take her to senior centers. She said she didn't want anything to do with those old people!

About four years ago she was driving home alone from my aunt's house when she encountered some construction. She panicked and flagged down the first two people she saw. When they said they would drive her home, she allowed one of the men to drive her car while the other followed. At that point, my brother and I were concerned that something must not be right, but Mom kept on driving even after that incident. My brother felt that if we took her license away she'd be completely dependent on us and he was panicking at that thought. Eventually she made some kind of mistake in the car that scared her. She never told us what it was. After that she stopped driving and was very sad because she had always been on the go. Her body was fine but her mind was going. Physically, she was more limber than I was at the time.

As far as symptoms go, I know my grandmother had dementia; she just sat in a chair, didn't know anybody, and didn't talk. She was around seventy-five, and that is about the age my mother's symptoms started.

The strangest thing that Mom did was put everything under the sofa. Her whole life revolved around this sofa, and so *everything* went under it. The sofa was on carpet and was difficult to move. I'd always have to get someone to help me move it to get all of Mom's stuff out. She had everything from food to socks to makeup under there. I couldn't understand why she was doing it and it drove me crazy. So, I spent a lot of time screaming at her, because my mother was very manipulative and argumentative. In her entire life, she never did anything anyone wanted her to do. As she got worse, these traits became more pronounced. She became very difficult and stubborn, refusing to dress or come to the table when she was asked to. There were a lot of times when I really couldn't tell if she was just being manipulative or she was really sick.

I took her to a psychiatrist about two years ago and he asked her a lot of questions. She was correct about the fact that she was married and how long she had been married, but mixed up on all the present-day information. The doctor told me that she had a type of dementia that progressed in stages. She seemed to be doing okay and then, all of a sudden, she'd be wearing the same clothes day after day. I was to later learn that she had multi-infarct dementia, a condition caused by a series of small strokes. This may cause rapid deterioration, but then the person seems to stay at the same level of functioning for quite a while before another stroke and another descent. The strokes are often imperceptible, occurring often in sleep.

For a while I was spending about five days a week at her house. My mother had shopped all her life and the house was filled with "stuff." I knew that if she had to go into a nursing home, we would have to get rid of a lot of things. Even though she would fight me, I would slip out with bags and take them to Goodwill. I did this for about two years. Then I had somebody come in to work at the house. That was horrible. It was a friend of a friend, a man who came highly recommended. But Mother would say that he did all these terrible things. She said he drank her orange juice, and made a lot of silly complaints. I remember thinking that there was no way to know who was telling the truth. And this was the only job this man had. My brother felt that having the aide come in to stay with Mother made everything harder because his presence seemed to set her off. Attempts to do anything beyond her regular pattern, activities like painting the cupboards and doing odd jobs around the house, made her very upset. She had always done everything herself: tiling floors, building cabinets, painting, and the like. My father would be out on the golf course. He never wanted any part of those things. She did it all, and he would bring people in and compliment her on her talents. So, ultimately, it was very hard for her to let anyone do anything for her that she thought she was able to do.

Then came the delusions. She started telling me about people having big parties downstairs and all the noise they were making. We explained that this was her house and nobody was having parties in her basement. It did no good. She gradually became more and more frightened of everything. We finally talked her into allowing a sitter to come in every day.

One of the funny incidents occurred one day when we were having lunch in a fast-food place. Mom noticed that some people near us had a little child with them. She kept saying, "What a cute little girl." I told her it was a little boy, but she just wouldn't let up and kept saying over and over, "Is that a little girl?" Finally, the man said, in front of everybody, "Would you like me to pull down his pants?!" I could have crawled under the chair!

Another time, on Easter, she came in after a walk around the block and said some kids had pushed and hurt her. I knew they hadn't. She had fallen and sprained her wrist. In the doctor's waiting room, where we waited to have a cast put on, Mother said to someone sitting nearby, "How do you like being in the minority?" It was another embarrassing moment. You never knew what was going to come out of her mouth.

Eventually, Mother had to come live with me because it was clearly unsafe for her to be alone anymore. One time when I came home, as I approached the back door, there was this awful smell. I didn't know what it was. Once in the kitchen, I started looking around and saw that the coffeepot was on and there was a yellowish liquid dripping down. I thought, "Oh no, she wouldn't—she couldn't!" Well, she had taken dog food instead of coffee grinds, and put it in the coffee filter! I never knew what the next day would bring.

One time, I called my mother from work to ask her to take out frozen vegetables and put them in the microwave. I had, up to that point, been able to manage her mostly by phone. This time, though, she didn't come back for the longest time and I heard all this rustling around. When she finally came back I said, "What in the world were you doing?" She said, "I was eating the vegetables you told me to eat." I said, "Oh no! I said HEAT, not EAT." She had eaten the vegetables right out of the freezer!

Now we have somebody with her during the day all the time. She's been functioning at about the same level for around four years now. The doctor says she just needs supervision. No doubt constant supervision will be needed later. We'll cross that bridge when we come to it. That's really all you can do.

Jean: We have quite a time with my mother-in-law. She was a child of the Depression and can't stand to see anything going to waste. She constantly takes things out of the garbage and puts them in the refrigerator! She'll take a piece of bread and pick the mold off of it. She keeps the house at around eighty-five degrees so everything molds quickly, but, if the tiniest bit is left over from a meal she saves it in a bowl in the refrigerator. Needless to say, the refrigerator is crammed full of leftovers. And it's hard to identify what's in the bowls because there will be things growing on them! We call them "specialties."

A few years ago I quit my job to stay home and take care of my father-in-law, who had become bedridden. We had a visiting nurse come in, and after a few visits, she told my husband that what was wrong with his mother was even worse than what was wrong with his father. We had been thinking that it was just the forgetfulness of old age, when, in fact, Mom didn't know what she was doing. And she was still driving! She would go to the store, and though it was only four blocks away, she'd be gone for four hours. She'd eventually find out where she was and make it home somehow.

When my father-in-law died we moved Mom in with us because we knew we couldn't leave her alone. We've had her now for two years, the longest two years of my life. The worst part was she became so paranoid. I stayed home with her for six months, but finally I had to get back to work. I couldn't take it any more. I'd go down to the mailbox on the corner and by the time I came back she had already locked the door and I couldn't get back in the house. She'd read all the bad reports in the paper and become frightened. She'd think burglars were coming to her house. It was one of the most difficult things to persuade her otherwise.

At first we made the mistake of staying home with her too much, and then one night when we didn't come home by eight o'clock as we usually did, she called the police and reported us missing. And they came! I guess it was because she seemed so frightened that they felt they had to investigate. She was always checking up on us, acting like we were still teenagers. And quite frankly, I don't know who she thinks I am, because half the time she thinks her son (my husband) is her husband. She sets the table for dinner and sets two places, one for him and one for her. I guess she thinks I'm the maid!

Last summer, my husband was away and I was out one evening visiting friends. Mom got their number from information somehow and called: "Do you know what time it is? It's time for you to be home!" I felt like crawling out of there! You know, the funniest thing was, people used to see my mother-in-law and talk to her for a couple of minutes and then say to me, "I don't know what you're talking about; she seems okay to me." So as Richard pointed out about his wife, people with dementia can really pull themselves together for a short time in many situations.

One of the most hilarious things that ever happened occurred when I returned a pair of slacks to a department store. The salesperson couldn't find the size I needed but said she was sure they could be found in another store and that she would call me when they came in. I left my home telephone number—crazy me. A couple of days later, they called and said to my mother-in-law, "We found Jean's pants." Well, she called me at work, yelling and screaming, "How could you lose your pants in a shopping mall? I'm going to call Bob and tell him what you did!" I had the phone to my ear, but my face must have shown some kind of emotion because everybody in the office was looking and laughing. To my mother-in-law, everything has something to do with sex. She preaches all the time!

On another occasion, I came home from work one evening and there were all these boxes and suitcases in the living room and by the front door. My husband was already home, but he was reading the paper, oblivious to it all. So I went out in the kitchen and made myself a cup of tea. Then I took a look in the suitcases and there were all my clothes! I said to my husband, "Didn't you happen to notice all the suitcases and boxes?" He said, "Oh, I thought it was just more of her craziness—I guess I didn't pay attention." She had packed everything I owned! Of course, when I confronted her she said, "I didn't do that!" She really acted as if she had no recollection of it.

"Does she sundown—get worse at night?" someone in the group asked.

Maybe—it's hard to tell. When we moved her in with us, we gave her our bedroom. The bedroom we occupy used to be the one she stayed in when she visited. Maybe she thought these were clothes of hers that she didn't wear anymore and she was packing them up. Who knows?!

While we're talking about nighttime occurrences, one time Mom got me up because she heard a puppy crying on the back porch. She went on so much about it that I finally went downstairs with her to check. I pretended to pick up the puppy, telling her I would put it in the basement so it would be warm. She was satisfied with that. You have to go along with them sometimes to get them past something they are obsessing about. And that kind of thing probably is more likely to happen at night.

I can really see, though, how being a little bit removed from the person, relationwise, helps to be more objective and makes it a little easier to cope. I started helping my mother-in-law take her bath once she reached the point where she didn't really know what to do in the tub. I started by just giving her directions. One time I gave her some simple instructions and left the bathroom. I heard the water running a bit too long and went to look in on her. She was sitting, fully clothed, on the bathroom floor next to the tub, with the water running, swishing at the water with one hand. I said, "Mom, you have to get undressed and get into the tub to take a bath." She said, "Oh, yeah." So I went out, thinking I really didn't need to watch, but she was in there a long time. When I went back in, she was sitting in the water, fully clothed! She just looked at me and said, "I know this isn't right, but I thought I would just sit here and wait until you came to check on me because I didn't know what I was supposed to do."

At that point, I knew I had to do it all myself—undress her, bathe her, and dry her off. Fortunately, she could still put her clothes on.

We had to disconnect the garbage disposal and toaster oven and take the knobs off the stove. One day I actually watched my mother-in-law take a clothespin that was in the kitchen and try to turn on the stove. It would have worked if I hadn't stopped her. But she couldn't figure out how to put the real knobs back on. We didn't have a hard time stopping Mom from driving but we had a rough time with the cooking. It was warming things up that was the problem. She'd put something on the stove and forget about it. She almost started many fires. Bill would come home for lunch every day when she was still staying alone, just to make sure she didn't try to cook herself something for lunch and burn the house down in the process! Once, I remember, we had brought her home a hamburger from a fast-food place and she didn't eat it right away. Instead, she put it in the refrigerator and then went to heat it up later. I was in the basement doing the laundry when I smelled something burning. I came up just in time to catch it before it became a real fire. She had put the hamburger in the toaster oven without taking the paper off!

(Someone piped up with, "Has anyone had someone burn something up in the microwave oven by putting a metal object in it?"

"Me! I did it myself," chuckled Richard. Everyone laughed.)

Mary: My mother was very independent-minded and got more so as she sensed the time living alone in her apartment coming to an end. We had talked for at least ten years about what would happen when she couldn't stay there anymore. When she was "with it" she was very clear about wanting to go to a nursing home that was right around the corner. Some of her friends in the apartment building had gone there. She would always say, "I'd like to go there if I can afford it." She didn't want to live with me before she got Alzheimer's, and after the dementia set in, it would have been impossible. She needs the structure of the nursing home and does very well in the day program for dementia patients.

One of the adventures we had during the last year she was in her apartment, when she was becoming more and more confused, was what I call the "sherry incident." Mother had never been much of a drinker. The only thing she liked was an occasional glass of cream sherry. To be cordial, she kept a bottle on hand to offer folks if they stopped by. It turned out that she was stopping by their apartments for a "sip," too. One late afternoon when I arrived, she was carrying around a cup of coffee with her. I mentioned that I didn't know she drank her coffee black and she told me right out that it wasn't coffee, it was sherry. She said it was her "little, before dinner toddy." This was midafternoon. So we had a talk about that. The cup had far more sherry in it than any toddy.

Mother was becoming more confused about what time of day it was and was pouring sherry to keep the cup half full, probably most of the afternoon and evening. At that point, I really think she thought each time she poured, it was the first time. Her short-term memory was just about gone. She was highly insulted that I dared to insinuate that she had a problem and was drinking too much. "Are you accusing me of being an alcoholic?" She told me indignantly that she knew she only had a little drink before dinner and before bed. She said she loved the taste of it and that I was just trying to take away her enjoyment. I found that she was stashing several 1.5-liter bottles in the closet. When confronted about it, she insisted that she liked to keep stocked up because her friends would drop by now and then and she liked to have something to offer them. To avoid a real scene, I waited until she was on the phone with her brother and took all the sherry out to my car. I searched and found more in another closet. When I left, I went straight to the store where I knew she was ordering it. They took the unopened bottles back, were very understanding about the situation, and promised not to send her any more sherry. They would just say they were out of it. Miraculously it worked and she wasn't able to call another store to try to get them to deliver. I had pictured myself having to contact every liquor store in town!

The very next day after the sherry incident, there came a "sherry-related incident." When I arrived for my daily visit after work, I found her door had been broken and repaired. It was easy to spot the repair because the wood was new and unpainted. One couldn't possibly miss it. By the time I got to the bottom of things, I found out that the police had had to break into the apartment the night before because Mother had fallen and could not get up. She had managed to pull the phone off a nearby table and instead of calling me, she dialed 911. The cover-up began the next day. She swore to secrecy the aide who came in three days a week to cook and do chores for her, saying she knew I would be very upset if I found out. She also told the lady next door, who had heard the police, not to tell me. I ran into that lady in the hallway and commented on the new piece of wood in the door and she told me everything. People were beginning to worry about Mother, as she was clearly at risk living there alone. She was not only getting more confused, but she had been on a continual "toot." And that, no doubt, had a lot to do with her fall. There had been some sherry left in an opened bottle, which I had not confiscated for fear that she would get too upset. It all got poured out that day. Thereafter, she only had a little glass at a family function or when we took her out to dinner. Fortunately, she never said anymore about it. She forgot!

Within a month we moved Mother into the nursing home. She hated to leave her apartment, which symbolized her independence, but she went willingly. Though my family was supportive, I went through the whole placement process virtually alone and it was quite a learning experience. All the people in the home were so good to her that she adjusted rather quickly. It has also made me realize that if you visit your loved ones frequently in the nursing home and monitor the kind of care they receive, you can free your mind of a lot of the negative myths about nursing homes and sleep well at night.

("You were lucky she didn't give you more trouble," someone remarked.

"I sure was," Mary admitted.)

They all sat around and talked for a few minutes about the blessing of being able to have some detachment in these situations. When you are right in the midst of these things, everyone agreed, it's hard to see the humor. Constantly "mopping up," both physically and emotionally, gets old very fast, when you are actually going through it. After a while the day can seem endless.

The group defined two kinds of detachment: One, involving

the passing of time that allows us to detach a bit from painful experiences, and the other involving the different levels of relationships that can exist between the Alzheimer's loved one and the caregiver (i.e., spouse, child, parent, in-law, and the like).

Needless to say, the closer the bond, the more difficult it is to see the forest for the trees. Perhaps it isn't until the metaphorical trees lose their leaves, symbolic of our allowing ourselves to open to others, that we know we are in a forest at all and can begin the inward journey that leads toward healing.

The session ended. Everyone seemed to feel good about sharing their humor, their stories, and ultimately their journeys.

Postscript

I have kept in touch with the people in the group from time to time. Some things have changed since we recorded the support-group session. Richard reports that he and his daughters have gone on with their lives. They are relieved that the "long good-bye" is over, but they have not forgotten. Martha, on the other hand, is not pleased with the facility in which her mother resides. Because of her job, and the distance to the nursing home, Martha can only visit once a week. She is trying to find a way to be more proactive in improving her mother's care. An update on Jean's mother is in the Postscript of the "Support Group II" chapter. Mary's mother still resides in the same nursing home. Visiting three or four times a week, Mary has found that frequent visits pay dividends. Her mother receives very good care. She wants people who cannot visit frequently because of other commitments to know that a good rapport with the staff is possible. Getting to know the staff when visiting and calling frequently can be effective, as well.

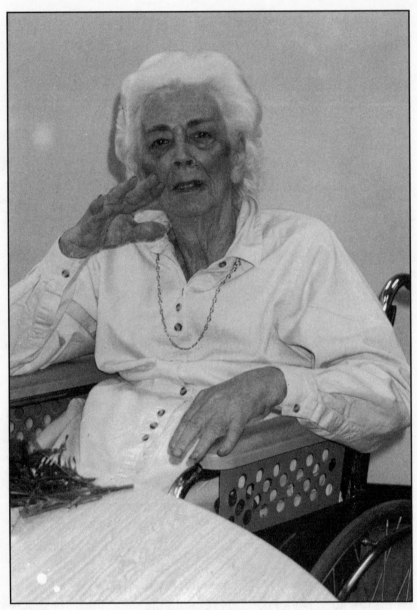

Ellen's mother, Mary Alice

Chapter 3

"I've Just Found Out I'm in Baltimore"

You met my mother in the first chapter.

Mother has been in a nursing home for over two years. In addition to the Alzheimer's, she is not able to walk except back and forth to the bathroom with a walker. She has severe osteoporosis, which keeps her limited to bed, her chair, or a wheelchair. She dozes in her chair frequently.

I work nearby and stop on my way home to be with her around dinnertime. Because I am her only child and because I truly want to, I try to visit her daily even if only for a short time. The look on her face when I approach makes it all worthwhile. It is a joyful expression and she is content while I am there. It seems as if her personality, boiled down to the level of the heart and soul, is pure love. When you ask her how she is, she is always "fine." Prior to the onset of dementia, that word was not in her vocabulary. She often had a complaint or negative comment to make. She had been somewhat of an invalid/recluse for much of her adult life and had a bit of an "attitude." In Mother's case,

57

dementia seems to have wiped out the bad memories and left only the good ones. Unusual? I'm sure it is, but it has actually happened that way. Strange as it may sound, her disposition has actually undergone a kind of improvement. She lives in the moment and seems to be happy most of the time. Surely she would laugh if she could remember her comment to me when she was in the very early stages of Alzheimer's. "I think I'm probably going to give you a hard time, Ellen, and I am sure sorry if I do." Actually, so far, I consider myself pretty fortunate.

One of the cutest and most amusing stories occurred when Mother was still able to use the phone. My number was written in big numbers taped to her phone. One day at work I decided to retrieve messages from my home answering machine. To my surprise, I heard the following: "Gee, I—I'm, so amazed—so overwhelmed that I called your number and you answered. This is your mother—and—and—I've just found out I'm in Baltimore. I can't get over that, Ellen, I really can't. I'm dying to see you! Call me when you can."

Mother has lived in Baltimore for thirty-six years but it is clear that the element of surprise is lurking everywhere when one has Alzheimer's. Some of the surprises are well received and some are not. During this message, however, Mother sounded like she was delighted with this new discovery.

To try to make a case for dementia being a blessing would obviously be ridiculous. All one can do is try to make the best of a bad situation. And it's important to remember that our own perceptions as caregivers are not always accurate. We are upset, overwhelmed, and frightened, to say nothing of the shadowy sense of fear that this may happen to us someday. As a result, much of what we do is not well thought out because we are so caught up in the negativity of the moment.

My point is this: we can't really know what our loved ones are experiencing. No matter how severe the dementia becomes, they are still human beings and still have brains, malfunctioning though they may be. Sometimes we have to check ourselves when we tend to become overly negative. It may be the human flair for drama that causes us to do this, but it's really important to try to keep things in perspective. Attending a support group is a good way to get objective feedback and overcome feelings of isolation.

Moreover, this is where faith and the power of positive thinking come in. Why can't we imagine that the Alzheimer's-afflicted loved one is basically no more unhappy than he or she was in general? It truly has been my observation, both personally and professionally, that the caregivers are often more unhappy than the patients. They are the ones who need coaching on where to find the "off button" when the negative thoughts start spinning around in their heads. Caregiving is something we will nearly all be called upon to do at some point in our lives. When a family begins to notice that one of its members is experiencing changes in mental status, the role automatically sets in to care for and pro-tect the loved one. A neighbor told me that her father had begun showing symptoms of dementia at around age sixty-nine. She said the family had experienced her dad coming down the stairs one morning and saying politely, "Can someone please point me in the direction of the kitchen?" He continued the same routine every morning thereafter. They realized he wasn't kidding. He was an extremely pleasant and polite man who never liked to interrupt anyone. It got so that he wouldn't even talk when a tele-vision commercial was on. He was experiencing the people on the screen as being right there in the living room, involved in the conversation. One day this gentleman left the house to take his daily walk around the block. He didn't come back. He was found by the police three days later sitting on the steps of a building, in the city, neat and clean. No one ever found out how he had sur-vived or how he had stayed so clean.

The point here is that the request for directions initially clued the family that something was amiss. The wandering off for three days thrust them headlong into caregiving roles. Also, this man clearly had an invisible means of support, what I call "hidden hands." Was it a guardian angel? To me, wonderful people who go out of their way to help others are human angels. Whatever the answer to this mystery, it was something good. That is the key . . . goodness and love. Again, love is what the Alzheimer's patient responds to. And in the final analysis, everything boils down to love. All of the suffering they go through, all of the suffering we, the caregivers, go through becomes one. And from that bond of suffering comes love in action, though love, the feeling, may not be present at all times. After all, it is not their fear but our own with which we have to deal. The roles have now reversed and child becomes parent, while parent becomes child. We laugh at, and with, our children as they come through the early milestones—crawling, walking, running, falling down. So, we go full circle when a parent is afflicted with Alzheimer's. Indeed, the adult becomes a child again and as children, we laugh when our parents laugh, even when we have a "boo-boo." The laughter heals us. And so it may be with dementia. Laughter can help ease the depression and anguish that accompany the sense of loss felt by the patient and the family.

I feel blessed by the fact that my mother has always had a good sense of humor. She likes to laugh a lot, even now, and frequently at herself, as she tries to say something and is aware of how wrong it is coming out. She recognizes the twisted sentence or mispronounced word and repeats it, laughing and saying, "Did you hear what I said?!" That may only be, however, because she was somewhat of an aficionado of the English language all her life. Her verbal social graces will probably be with her until the end. A patient who is a former athlete, on the other hand, may be able to walk until the end, and may enjoy pacing. We "are" what we "do" during our productive lifetimes and it gives us pause to imagine what we would be like, and what our families would have to cope with, if we became afflicted with Alzheimer's ourselves.

I can't help thinking often about the kind of mind my mother had, her incredible memory that was far superior to mine. She learned to concentrate at an early age due to an excellent education and having the good fortune of being a member of a family of constant readers. It seems the world we live in today bombards us with so much stimulation that life has become a continuous multimedia event, moving at an ever-faster pace. It's a wonder anyone can concentrate. Now, when referring to her memory, Mother will say, "It's all just like a big blank!" One day she quipped, "I guess if there were anything important to know, you or someone would tell me."

Mother's world was very different, and her memories of that world are scattered, but still more or less intact. When she talks about something from the past and gets stuck, I will often suggest the way it might have been. She looks at me and says, "Yes, that's close enough, and how come you're so smart and I'm getting to be so dumb?!" Then she chuckles and says, "I can't remember anything anymore, you know, so there's really no use asking." One day as she caught herself looking in the medicine cabinet for a towel, she quipped, "If you are worried about my sanity, you have good reason to be." She still has insight and can be very philosophical. Those are her strong points.

One of the last outings we had as a family before my aunt died was a visit to a favorite restaurant. I ordered soft-shell crabs for both Mother and Auntie Peg. It had always been their favorite. When the plates were put in front of them they both had the same puzzled expression on their faces. Then they started whispering to each other and laughing. They were looking around at the plates the rest of us had, more normal-looking fare, like meat and potatoes or pasta. It took a few minutes for us to figure out why they were giggling and whispering. Finally, Mother said, "You all have dinners and we have these spiders on our plates. Do you really expect us to eat them?" We tried not to laugh, but failed, as we realized what was happening. Neither of them had any idea what the soft-shell crabs were or what to do with them. I carefully explained as we cut them into manageable bites. It did no good. They were having none of it. We ordered them soup and sandwiches and everyone was happy!

In *The 36-Hour Day*, coauthored with Peter Rabins, M.D., Nancy Mace says, "Clearly, for some patients, some of the time, having dementia is not synonymous with suffering. We caregivers and health care professionals can make a difference in whether such people suffer with their illness or whether they are comfortable and able to enjoy moment to moment. These success stories are rare. They are far outnumbered by stories of patient suffering and family suffering." She goes on to say she feels our obligation is to learn what we can do to improve the quality of the lives of both patient and family.

That is most specifically what we are about here. By sharing the story of my mother's and my journey, I am hoping to prove that it doesn't have to be all bad. Our story leans toward the "success story" side, but I am living it as I am writing it, so who knows what the outcome will be. And how would she and my aunt feel about being in this book? I have to believe that they both would approve. Both would want to contribute to the process of finding a cure for Alzheimer's. My aunt worried about getting it as she was descending into the labyrinth. Being the person she was, I think it broke her heart, and she would want to do anything possible to keep anyone else from having to go through it.

Mother, on the other hand, was never aware that it was Alzheimer's. Her short-term memory got so bad, so quickly, that even if the idea entered her mind, it just as quickly fled. That was really a mercy. What seems like another blessing is that Mother really likes TV. It serves well as company for her because she can't read anymore. She can still read something out loud, a sentence or two. But, a book is now beyond her capability, as each page would be immediately forgotten as she read it, making it impossible to make any sense of the story. Her fondness for TV was expressed recently when she told me that she thinks "television is wonderful and the best invention ever." She said, "You know, I learn a lot from it." She's usually referring to the commercials, which she gets a kick out of—lots of movement and color. She is positively wild about babies and every time a baby comes on the screen she says, "Now that is the most beautiful baby I think I've ever seen." Every single baby—bar none!

There are lots of memorable moments that involved Mother and Auntie Peg. When they were both becoming forgetful, each would think the other was much worse off and make such comments as, "You already told me that five times!" The other would say to me, "She must think I'm some kind of a dummy."

In my aunt's apartment one night after dinner, she and Mother sat in the dark bedroom, looking out over the lights of the city. I was reading in the living room, when I heard them start to debate about "what was that bright light in the sky." And it was moving! Remarks were made such as, "You know, that thing up in the sky that whirls around." "Yes, and sometimes the police are in them." The discussion went on for about ten minutes and neither of them could come up with the word. I listened for a while and then went in and said "helicopter." They laughed and laughed!

Another time, shortly before my aunt's death, when I had taken Mother over to visit her, they attempted to have a conversation. Auntie Peg's ability to speak had all but left her. She could only mumble a few things. Usually anything that came as a response to something said by someone else was completely irrelevant to the topic. I was sitting with them and Mother kept trying to pull an answer out of Auntie Peg. I finally muttered something like "Don't keep questioning her, she doesn't understand." Mother looked highly indignant and stated loudly, "I not only have a crazy sister, I have a crazy daughter, too!" I tried not to laugh—too hard.

Dr. Oliver Sacks, author of *Awakenings* and *The Man Who Mistook His Wife for a Hat,* said, "In dementia, or other such catastrophes, however great the organic damage and human dissolution, there remains the undiminished possibility of reintegration by art, by communion, by touching the human spirit. . . . A person does not consist of memory alone. He/she has feeling, will, sensibilities, moral being—matters of which neuro-psychology cannot speak." I have found that music is a wonderful tool of communication. Just sitting with Alzheimer's patients and watching them respond is rewarding. They especially love the songs from their early years and can usually remember some of the words that go with the tune.

For the caregiver, keeping spirits up, "accessing mirth," and sometimes downright laughter (be it a little hysterical or not) are the avenues to reintegration into something that feels like normal. I believe that a very fine quality of being human is that we can laugh in the midst of disaster and, sometimes, even joke in the middle of a crisis. It is a protective device that helps get us through. Whistling in the dark is an age-old tonic.

Most of the literature I researched emphasized that the caregiver experience is characterized by the adjustment of the Alzheimer's patient and his/her family to the illness. We cannot characterize it as a positive experience, but some of us can be lucky enough to have not such a bad go of it. My children feel that we have been fortunate in that Auntie Peg's case didn't go on terribly long and that Mother seems pretty content, at least for now.

Postscript

The good news about Mother is that she now has her very own "most beautiful baby." Her great-grandson, Tommy, was born the summer of 1997. Now she doesn't have to see babies only on TV. She is very responsive to Tommy and he to her. She may not understand the concept of the relationship, but she knows he is someone important to her. A large picture of him sits on her bureau. Recently, I pointed to the picture and said, "This is your great-grandson, you know." Somewhat garbled, but intelligible to me, she responded, "Now, tell me again how this came about." I said, "Lynne had a baby, remember?" Mother looked at me and said, excitedly and clearly, "She did? When?!"

So! You won't be surprised to hear, once again, that there can be something new and different every day in the lives of even the most seriously afflicted Alzheimer's patients.

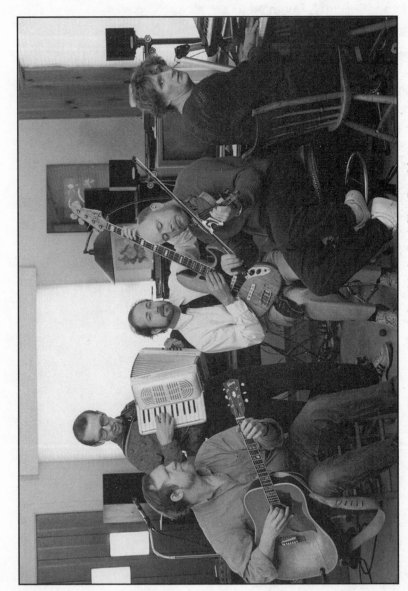

Tommy Thompson (far left) with the Red Clay Ramblers

Chapter 4

Tommy Thompson

This is the story of Tommy Thompson, singer and banjo player with the Red Clay Ramblers, a group that has performed both on and off-Broadway for the past twenty years.

One morning, during the time that I was collecting stories for this book, I heard Tommy being interviewed on the radio. It was classic serendipity. Through good fortune, I was able to get in touch with Tommy in Carrboro, North Carolina. From the very first phone meeting we had, I liked Tommy, and knew he was someone I wanted to include in the book. Though he has been a celebrity for many years, he is a very generous person and agreed to be involved. He was interested in making his own special contribution to finding the cure for his diminishing capacity as well as helping others.

In the spring of 1995, at the age of fifty-eight, it had been a year or so since Tommy had undergone medical testing and been told that he had something resembling early-onset Alzheimer's disease. In 1993, Tommy said he had noticed that he would play an odd note now and then when performing with the Red Clay Ramblers on

Broadway. He was bothered by these "bloopers" because he is a perfectionist and felt it interfered with his performance.

Tommy had been playing the banjo with the band since he helped form it in 1972. In 1994, he was the last original member of the Red Clay Ramblers and he was leaving the group. The more he talked about it, the more nostalgic he became, so we went back to the beginning.

Born in West Virginia in 1937, Tommy's love for music began when he was very young. He had a good sense of pitch and could sing all the radio (and later, TV) commercials. He bought a guitar and chord chart and taught himself to play. Then, he saw someone playing a banjo and became interested in becoming a banjo player.

Tommy graduated from Kenyon College in Ohio, in 1959. He married his high school sweetheart and joined the Coast Guard with plans to support a family. His Coast Guard duties required occasional visits to bayou country, and there he was introduced to the noble crawfish and to the sound of Cajun music. In 1963, he entered the graduate program at the University of North Carolina in Chapel Hill. At that point, he divided his time between a five-string banjo and academia, specializing in drop-thumb clawhammer and conceptual analysis. Two years later, he formed the Hollow Rock String Band, a group devoted to the old-time dance tunes of the southern mountains.

Moving ahead to 1971, Tommy won the World Champion Old Time Banjo Contest at Union Grove, North Carolina. During that same year, Barbara, his ex-wife, was killed in an auto accident. By this time, Tommy had a five-year-old son, also named Tom, from a different relationship. Tommy freely admits that his fatherhood was overshadowed, at times, by his developing career in music. In 1972 he helped organize the Red Clay Ramblers. The band started out as a three-man string band devoted to styles of early-recorded country music. They added piano and horns and reached beyond to gospel, Celtic, and blues. They even played fox-trots. Two years later, the Ramblers joined the cast of *Diamond Studs*, a musical about Jesse James, and spent the first seven months of 1975 performing off-Broadway in New York City. The musical instruments in the band included a banjo, a tuba, fiddles, trumpets, drums, and penny whistles. The sounds that were produced by the various mixing of these instruments were magical. Currently, all albums produced by the group are put out by Sugar Hill Records in Durham, North Carolina.

Since their first tour in the fall of 1975, the Ramblers, now a five-man band, have traveled throughout the United States, Canada, Europe, the Middle East, and Africa. Tommy has composed many of the songs performed and recorded by the Red Clay Ramblers and other artists. His creative credits for the theater include *Life on the Mississippi* (1981), *John Proffit* (1984), *A Lie of the Mind* by Sam Shepard (1985), *Earrings* (a theatrical adaptation of Lee Smith's novel, *Oral History*) (1986), *The Merry Wives of Windsor, Texas* (a horse opera) (1988), and *Savages*, a play by John Justice (1992).

Tommy tells some good stories about the various experiences of the Red Clay Ramblers. One evening, thirteen or fourteen years ago, the group was cramped in a small orange van full of guitars and "what-all," traveling southeast from Calgary. They had driven straight through the first night and through the next day. After being on the road for two days straight, they were hankering for a cheap motel. A good sleep would allow just enough time for them to play the last scheduled concert two days hence at Northern Iowa University. They were having an argument because Tommy had promised the local public radio station on campus that they would arrive a day early to do a live broadcast (for no pay). Tommy supports public radio stations partly because they provide most of the group's airtime. Besides, he thought the radio exposure would help promote their concert. Some in the group said, "We don't go without sleep to give free shows. Exposure is what people die of." They were tired and it had been a foolish promise. But, nevertheless, all agreed that it was too late to break it. So they pressed on for twenty-two more hours, arrived at the station minutes before airtime, "glum and

smelly," and gave them a show. It turned out to be well worth the
trouble. The station dealt with the group's tardy and disgruntled
arrival with friendly efficiency. They had pulled in a small,
enthusiastic audience of Red Clay Rambler fans, the sound rein-
forcement was fine, and somewhere out there, in the middle of
Iowa, the great playwright Sam Shepard was listening.

That all happened in 1982 and Sam was on location for the
filming of the movie *Country*. In the fall of 1985, he was in New
York, directing the premier production of his new play, *A Lie of the
Mind*. It is his practice to mix music with theater, and this time he
intended to use the recorded singing of "two 'high lonesome' prim-
itives," Skip James and Roscoe Holcomb. For some reason, he
changed his mind and decided that only live music would properly
serve the show. He remembered the Red Clay Ramblers. Somebody said he noticed the band's name on an old *Diamond Studs*
poster. Phone calls were made, deals were discussed, and Tommy
and another member of the group flew to New York to meet the
"man with the right stuff." Tommy claims their first meeting
together "was blessedly comfortable and ordinary—just a roomful
of extraordinary actors drinking bad coffee out of Styrofoam cups."

Tommy felt that sometimes Sam Shepard seemed more at
home with the Ramblers than with the cast. He is a musician
himself, and knows the language. "Of course the group was
bending over backwards with tractability," Tommy adds. Sam
has a good sense of how a roughed-in piece of music will eventually work when it has been refined and placed. Tommy says he
looks for the emotional content of a scene or moment, and avoids
"character themes" and dramatic clichés. Sam asked the Ramblers to write or find songs that made no direct reference to the
play's action or characters. He wanted music that felt old, music
that would carry his notion that the same absurd and dreadful
conflicts have plagued families forever. Often as not, he would
ask for a song or melody that, instead of supporting an actor's
lines, would undercut it with irony. The group made some pretty

good music for *A Lie of the Mind*, much better than it would have been without Sam's intuitive artistry.

The show opened in early December of 1985. After the second performance, Sam met the group backstage to say good-bye. The usual compliments and thanks were exchanged, and then, as he was about to go, he said that they would work together again. He said to them, "We'll do a film." Tommy remarks, "That is a sentence that a person can say softly, with his mouth barely open." After a couple of years they began to wonder if he had really said it.

Good as his word, in the fall of 1988, the movie *Far North* was released, written and directed by Sam Shepard. Once again, Sam had gone to his producers and said, "These are the guys who are doing the score. Period." The movie *Silent Tongue* was made later, also written and directed by Shepard. This time, the Ramblers were actually in the film, on screen.

"Those were good times," Tommy reflects.

But now, times have changed and the "intruder" has come into his life. Naturally, the tentative diagnosis of Alzheimer's is devastating to Tommy and his family. But Tommy's positive outlook on life and his philosophical nature are seeing them through. This one-time philosophy teacher sees what is happening as "part of the human comedy," about which he could have done absolutely nothing. He admits to getting angry, at times, about his diminishing capacity, but feels that as long as he has projects to look forward to he doesn't worry about it. He says he feels he has now moved to another stage of what life is all about. Grateful to have had a professional career on Broadway for over twenty years, he says with a chuckle, "I don't have to be wonderful all my life."

Tommy has been taking Cognex (Tacrin), the only drug approved at this time for treating his memory problems. It has some side effects, so he went off it for a week. He now realizes that that was a mistake. There was a noticeable difference in his ability to remember things and it took a couple of weeks back on the medication to get to the point of receiving the maximum benefit again.

I really felt honored talking to this man. He is a very engaging person, with a great sense of humor. Tommy even describes himself as lucky because he was blessed with a sunny disposition. One day, while we talked on the phone, the radio was on in the background and he heard that Burl Ives had just died. They were playing one of his songs and we both stopped to listen. Burl Ives had been a hero of Tommy's and he describes his own voice as somewhat similar. He also says he used to be a much bigger man until he decided he didn't want to be that "big" anymore. What worked for him was walking. He describes himself as six foot one and a hundred and ninety-five pounds. Tommy admits, with candor, that he is a good singer. It is a given that he loves music and at the present time, he gets together with friends once a week for a jam session.

Tommy's daughter, Jessica, is getting married soon. His son, Tommy, is in the army. Both are doing well and that gives Tommy a sense of happiness and peace. His comment was, "They are both hunky and dory," followed by a chuckle and, "Sorry, I just ramble on." He added that now when he cries, it is tears of joy because of his wonderful children, wonderful friends, and his love for music. Tommy feels gratitude for what he feels are many blessings.

Jessica told me she admires the way her father is dealing with his illness. She is a special education teacher who works with emotionally challenged children. She, no doubt, has that special kind of patience needed to help her father navigate his troubled waters. Next year, she will be teaching the learning disabled, which she says will be a welcome change. Though she doesn't live nearby, Tommy wears a bracelet with her telephone number on it, in the event he should ever get lost. Jessica visits her father frequently and helps him with such chores as paying bills and planning details of the trips he takes. Tommy has friends all over the country and has visited friends in Florida and Seattle recently. He finds planning the details of taking a trip and maneuvering through airports a real challenge.

Jessica is honest enough to say that she and her brother didn't see as much of their father during their childhood as they would have liked. His career was taking off and there was a lot of travel involved. She had a heartwarming story to tell about Tommy that occurred within the past year. Last Christmas they heard about a church charity that would provide clothes for children. Tommy's wish was to go out and buy a pair of blue jeans for a six-year-old boy. Jessica thinks he remembered how much he would have liked a new pair of blue jeans when he was six.

Tommy has deep spiritual values, though he doesn't describe himself as religious. He takes the long view of things, even though he says his years of teaching philosophy were very technical and did not necessarily lead him to becoming philosophical. Tommy is grateful for the life he has lived to this point and seems to have an upbeat attitude about the future, albeit having to cope with the burden of a memory-disabling illness. He is very courageous.

What could be more uplifting than talking to a man like Tommy Thompson? Indeed, in my book, he is a hero.

Postscript

At this point in Tommy's life, the summer of 1998, he is still living in his apartment. He now goes out to a day program. Jessica is married and lives nearby and his son, Tommy, now out of the army, also lives near enough to see his father weekly. Tommy is taking a new medication, Aricept, to improve his memory. It has very few side effects.

Tommy's children have been wonderful in helping to develop this chapter. They are also gifted, with talents including singing, writing, photography, and language. They both feel grateful to their creative parents for their own artistic abilities. One of Tommy's greatest pleasures now is helping his daughter with her singing. Music and his family are still the greatest joys of his life. And most of all, Tommy Thompson is still blessed with a buoyant spirit.

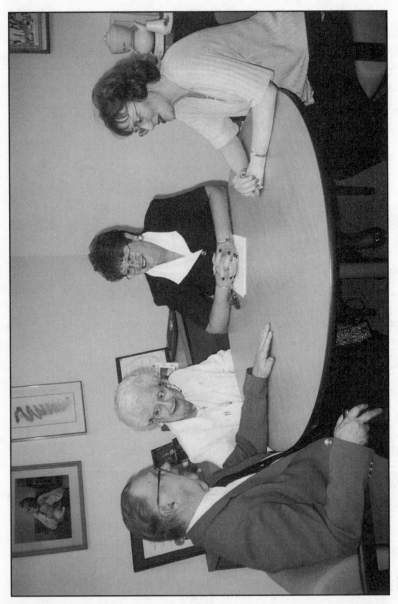

From left: Tom, Evelyn, Jean, and Ellen

Chapter 5

Support Group II

"Hold Your Head Up, Charlie Brown"

A second visit to the Alzheimer's Association many months after the first support group meeting resulted in the following transcript. One of the same caregivers who attended the first group returned to update us on her mother-in-law and two new caregivers joined us.

Ellen: My reason for coming today is once again to talk to people about some of their more positive experiences in taking care of Alzheimer's patients, which include their mothers, fathers, spouses, in-laws, etc. I have had an amazing experience with my own mother.

Nancy Mace in *The 36-Hour Day* (coauthored by Peter Rabins, M.D.), talked about the fact that there are success stories. They may be very few and far between, but I think we need to build on that. There are a lot of caregivers who are shut in and have no access to support groups—they are unable to attend because there is no one to take over the job for them. They are often lonely and depressed. My mission is to bring the support group to them.

75

They may be in the middle of the crisis and not be able to see any humor or bright side to anything. Reading this book is not necessarily going to turn the light on for them instantly, but it might help them to feel that they are not alone and that they are sharing in these stories. So I want to hear about your journeys.

Evelyn: I have a husband and a sister-in-law who both have Alzheimer's disease. When I first started taking care of Helen, she lived in Richmond. There was one particular weekend when we were trying to get her acclimated to her new surroundings. She had moved to a retirement community in a different part of town. I had a map and was trying to get my husband, John, to veer into the right lane to enter a shopping mall. We finally got over. Then it suddenly dawned on me that Helen was recovering from a fractured vertebra, so she couldn't walk very much. We'd have to let her off at the front door, then I would go with John to park the car. But Helen would probably wander off—so I would lose her. If I were to get out with Helen and let John go park the car, we wouldn't lose John, because he was still able to park and find his way to the front door of the store, but we would lose the car. He wouldn't remember where the car was by the time we came out. If I were to leave John and Helen and I park the car, I wouldn't lose the car, but I might lose Helen and John. It was like a riddle—the riddle we knew when we were kids, about the fox, the goose, and the bag of grain and how to get them all across the river. When something is funny like that, it's hard to know quite what to do. If you are going to laugh, the Alzheimer's loved one isn't going to know why you are laughing. So I was sitting there, and it was not a bit funny, but I could have roared with laughter. And as luck would have it, there was a place to park near the front door, so I didn't have to solve the riddle.

On another occasion, John and Helen were in the front seat and I was in the back seat with the map so we wouldn't get lost. The windshield was fogging up and I knew you had to push the lever to the right to defog. I told Helen what to do but she touched everything but the lever. "No, over to the left," and she didn't know what left was. "It's up a little," but she didn't know up from down. The windshield was getting foggier and foggier. So I thought, "Okay, I'll have to lean over the front seat." So I started leaning over the seat and I suddenly thought, "What am I doing?" I was perched there with my middle getting cut in half, as I finally was able to push the lever over, and the window immediately began to defog. But then it began to get cold, because it was on air-conditioning. Helen started to complain of the cold. "I'm cold—where's this cold air coming from?" In order to get heat, I'd have had to get under John's elbow, and I decided, "No, Helen, you're just going to have to be cold. We're not going to be in the car very much longer—you'll be fine." She fussed for the rest of the trip.

Ellen: You know, when you say they don't know why you're laughing, you have to be careful. I've found that quite often, if you laugh, then they laugh, and the atmosphere lightens up. It depends on the stage they are in. If it's in the early stage they could question your mirth and perhaps be insulted. So it's a delicate balance, no doubt about it. But we also must find a way to "access mirth" for ourselves, to go within, turn things around, become a magician, and get a different perspective. These little stories you are telling, Evelyn, are wonderful. But some folks might get bogged down emotionally and say, "Oh no, this is a drag, she can't even push a lever anymore." And then it's really easy to get lost in "other-pity," "self-pity," or just a "pity-party," in general.

Evelyn: There are circumstances that are not funny, at the time, to the caregiver. But later, you remember the event, and you realize how ridiculous you were, and how it really was funny. I often say in the midst of something that's driving me right up the wall, "In another week I'll be able to look back on this and laugh."

Ellen: Yes, and that is a perfect example of accessing the strength and the grace needed to get through.

Tom: My mother-in-law, Clara, came to live with us a number of years ago and it took a while to understand how bad off she was. One day, my wife left for a meeting and I gave her a hug and kiss good-bye. My mother-in-law was only sometimes cognizant, at this stage, of who we were, individually. Occasionally, I was her daughter and her son-in-law at the same time. I was her son-in-law more often than my wife was her daughter, because, of course, she would remember her daughter as a little girl. A grown woman couldn't possibly be her daughter. She wasn't old enough to have a daughter that age! Clara is eighty-six now, she was about seventy-eight then.

One day, we were sitting on the sofa with the TV on. I don't know whether she was watching or not, but she was sitting there quietly. At this point I had figured out that she confused me with about half a dozen different people and my wife with at least that many different people. So, when she saw me kiss my wife (who to her was this woman) good-bye, she nudged me with her elbow and said, "Tom, I think you ought to know that it's not wise to have a wife and a girlfriend at the same time."

As a follow up to this, about a week or two later, she had one of those rare, lucid moments, an hour or two, when there was absolutely nothing wrong with her mind. Her memory was perfect. She remembered who we were. She remembered getting very sick and coming to live with us. She remembered running away and being picked up by the police. So I said, "Clara, do you remember poking me and telling me that it's not wise to have a wife and a girlfriend at the same time?"

"Yeah."

So I said, "How come you didn't tell her?"

She said, "I didn't want to make any trouble for you!"

I asked her if she remembered the night the police picked her up when she wandered away.

"Oh yeah, they were nice."

She had been wandering on a busy main drag at rush hour.

She had to use the restroom and went into a local establishment. That's when the waitress figured out something was amiss and notified the police. Since we had also alerted them, it was fairly easy for them to put two and two together, and it wasn't long before we had her back. She told us that she and a few nice men were having a beer together and they brought her back home. The police quickly defended their "on duty honor" to say they weren't allowed to drink on duty. Of course, we knew that the beer part was wrong, since she had been picked up at an ice cream store. This was all a while back. She is now in the end stages of the disease and on home hospice care. It could be days or a couple of months, at most, until she will be going home to heaven.

Ellen: Does she communicate at all now? Is she totally bedridden?

Tom: As an engineer, you realize that it can be the tiniest amount of anything and it still exists, so "Does she communicate still?" I'd have to say "Yes." For example, just the other day when I was trying to get some food and water into her, she mumbled a little bit. I think that she is in greater internal stress than normal right now, because whenever she is under stress she seems to be a little bit more lucid and have a little longer-term memory. So I tried giving her some pureed vegetable soup, which she had eaten reasonably well before, and she muttered, barely intelligibly, "I don't want it." But I continued to try, pouring a tiny bit on her tongue. With that, she sprayed it back at me and said loudly, "I said I didn't want it!"

Ellen: It is amazing how lucid they can seem at the end. My aunt had been suffering for two years with Alzheimer's. It struck right after her hip replacement. She had been an extremely active, independent person, high functioning for eighty-three, and knew something terrible was happening to her. So, she just gave up and then went downhill very fast. In the hospital, she had a stroke and the day before she died she became quite lucid. She knew who the family members were, names and all, and was generally more responsive. It's almost as if there are little "cosmic rays" that light up the brain, especially near the end.

Evelyn: Every time you say they don't remember, they make a liar out of you. My mother-in-law also had Alzheimer's. One time I was going to a church retreat down in Virginia. The family insisted she wouldn't know I was gone. I was gone five days. When I came back, it was like she was my child and I had to go to the nursing home to see her right away. My family said to wait; no hurry. But I went anyway and when I got to her bedside, she looked up at me and said, clearly, "Evelyn, don't ever leave me again." I promised her I wouldn't. It was an easy promise because she was dying and she only lived another several months. She had mini-strokes toward the end. There was one time when we called her son in Massachusetts and he came with his wife and five children. I decided to take the day off and let them be with her that day. At three o'clock in the afternoon I felt I had to be there and went anyway. She had grandchildren sitting on her bed, her son and daughter-in-law next to her, and she looked at me and said, "Oh Evelyn, I've been waiting all day for you." My sister-in-law said, "We came four hundred fifty miles and all you want is Evelyn." They get such an attachment to the one they see the most. I think there is a safety factor involved.

Ellen: I think also that as the capacity to remember diminishes in Alzheimer's, the ability to relate to many different people or to even know who they are diminishes concurrently.

Jean: I often think my mother-in-law wishes I would drop off the face of the earth, so she could be with her son. But when I go away for a few days and come back, you'd think I had been gone a year, she is so happy to see me.

Evelyn: You spell safety to her. When I go to visit my sister-in-law in the nursing home, she still knows who I am and just lights up. It's as if she's thinking, "You're here, you're here." That is why I had to stop going to the support group in the nursing home. I would leave John up in the room with her. He was fine and nobody minded that he was there. He didn't cause any extra problems. But she would keep saying, "Where is Evelyn, where is Evelyn?" John wouldn't remember where I was, but he would figure, "Well, she's somewhere" and was not unhappy about it. He would go looking for me down the corridor. One time, when I got back to the room, Helen was sobbing uncontrollably in the nurse's arms. She took one look at me and she said, "Oh, you're all right." Since John wasn't able to tell her where I was, I guess she figured something must be wrong, that I was lost or gone.

Ellen: So Evelyn, you have had three bouts with Alzheimer's —your husband, your mother-in-law, and your sister-in-law.

Evelyn: Yes, and because John and his sister knew about their mother, they began to pick up on their memory loss very early. John was very philosophical about it. You can't do anything about it, so why fuss over it? I remember a time, my sister, who was a gourmet cook, gave me a recipe for a wonderful chicken dish, but it didn't have any amounts listed, so I had to do some guessing. I said, "Oh my goodness, this is never going to taste as good as Barbara's."

"Don't worry, Honey," John said, "I won't remember what Barbara's tasted like anyway."

John had been very ill as a young man, and had almost lost his life. I also had some very serious ailments at about the same time. You gain a perspective that I don't think you ever lose. You recognize that there are some things that you can do something about and there are some things that you just can't. And you will make your life miserable if you continue to beat your head against the wall about it. So John was very easy to get along with, and still is pretty easy. He hates it when I help him shave, though. I put cream around his nose, on his upper lip, and on his chin because it is so dry. And I joke about how "women have their problems, but having to shave your face every day of your life from the time you're a teenager must be a pain." Just this morning, I started singing, "You are my sunshine, my only sunshine," so he had to break up and laugh over that. I said, "Oh Honey, I love you so much and you love me too, don't you?" And he said gruffly, "Yes, I do." He's not very verbal, and much of the time there is a lot of nonverbal communication going on the way it does anyway, between people who have been married for so many years. In the morning, he's up first, and I say, "Honey, let's get the curtains open and let the sunshine in. How are you today? Are you well?" And he'll say, "I'm yes." I hug him and say, "I'm so glad you're yes, it would be awful if you were no."

I'm the original Pollyanna. I was on crutches for many years. I have crutches in the basement, and when I look at them, I am so happy that I don't need them, just like Pollyanna was glad when she took the crutches out of the missionary barrel. In the first of the series of stories about Pollyanna, she picks out a pair of crutches and says, "Oh, I'm so glad I don't need these crutches!" She could always find something to be glad about. So when people call me Pollyanna, they don't know how true it is, that I'm awfully glad I don't need those crutches anymore.

Ellen: How long has it been since you first noticed signs of impairment and then until John was diagnosed?

Evelyn: I first saw signs, only in retrospect, when I thought, "Why is John not redoing the little bedroom after we've had the roof repaired? And why isn't he painting the bathroom and the basement when they both need painting? Why do I have to push him to do these things?" That was about 1986. By the following year, I realized that the reason he wasn't doing these things was that they were too complicated for him.

Jean: My father-in-law reached a point where he realized he couldn't do things, such as drive or handle his finances. He was very good about it. My mother-in-law still does not understand why she can't drive. We still let her keep her checkbook and she writes checks to everyone who sends her mail and she is on everybody's list. She gets mail from these lobbying organizations that are talking about Medicare benefits and Social Security and she writes them checks. Fortunately she does not write them for large amounts; it will usually be only five or ten dollars. But when we go over her checkbook every month, it's nothing for her to have given five hundred dollars. So lately, we've been trying to reason with her. "You know, Mom, you wrote three checks to the same people this month." "Oh, I did?" So now she just puts the mail on the table by the front door, because we told her we don't want her to fall down the front steps. Then we'll take it to the mailbox when we go out. Now we check through the mail and a few are shoved in our pockets on the way. She hears the mailbox close and is happy.

Evelyn: This happened to us one year. We had always been supporters of the symphony and sent in our generous one-time check. Well, John sent it in two more times. So the following year, they expected that much or more. So I told them that they had received three times what was meant to be and this year I was going to have to pull in my horns. They were very understanding. If John could have saved the environment single-handedly, he would have done it. Every month there were checks to so many different organizations that I really had to start telling these people, "I'm awfully sorry, but I'm the giver now and things have changed."

Jean: It's really been one of the more difficult things with my mother-in-law, because she reads these letters and they all sound so real, and you can't reason with her. You can't convince her that this is not Medicare canceling her insurance. This is a lobbying organization. That doesn't mean anything to her. She says, "Jean, it says right here, my benefits are canceled."

I say, "Mom, your benefits are with Blue Cross. Does that say Blue Cross on the letterhead?" That's when she gets really feisty and adamantly declares, "Well, it's my money!"

Evelyn: Then there are the problems with the telephone solicitors. One night a man was coming to demonstrate a safety system, complete with the buzzer worn on the body. I think this man had already spent his commission, that's how certain he was we were going to buy it. I sat there trying to figure out how we were going to say no to him. He said, "Your husband thinks this system sounds wonderful."

"It may sound wonderful but we don't have that kind of money," I responded. "If John is out mowing the lawn and suddenly he collapses, we live in a row house development and someone's going to see him." There were several of these appointments set up, and, of course, when I asked John if he had made them, he didn't remember.

Jean: Many home-improvement people come to the house and my mother-in-law would give them cash to fix whatever it was she needed done. So now we don't let her have a whole lot of cash. There may always be twenty or twenty-five dollars around, but other than that, she doesn't know of any other cash in the house. People would come in and tell her that the roof was going to fall in or the windows weren't safe. This feeds her paranoia that someone is going to break in. We've limited her giving money away like that.

Evelyn: But she was letting them in the house. It's lucky nothing ever happened.

Jean: I think it's because of the fact that they never know when someone is coming to the house, because if they had been watching, there is always someone stopping in. We have people coming in from the church to see her, neighbors stopping by, and Dick sometimes comes home for lunch. So if anyone is trying to watch the house to catch a pattern, it's kind of difficult. I guess that's what has protected us.

Ellen: At our last meeting, your mother-in-law would sometimes call the police if you and your husband were not home when she thought you should be. How is that going?

Jean: That's our biggest problem. We really can't go out at night at all. She doesn't like to have anyone stay with her. But we have arranged to place her in a home for respite care for a week while we visit my mother in Florida. Now I'm getting guilty feelings from the other side of the family. My mother fell and broke her ankle in October and had to go for rehab. I haven't even been able to get down to see her yet. I've realized that while I'm taking care of my mother-in-law, there is a good possibility that my mother could go first. And I don't know that I can live with that kind of guilt.

Ellen: This is a perfect example of the process of looking at the entire family system and not allowing the "identified patient" to take up all the time, attention, emotion, and energies. It isn't fair to anyone.

Jean: What has surprised me is that my mother-in-law is willing to do this at all. At first we were going to have a woman come and stay with her but when Mom spoke with her on the phone, she decided that she didn't want that arrangement. The next option was that a woman from church offered to have my mother-in-law stay with her. But she said she didn't want to impose on anyone else. So, that idea was out. We said that we just wouldn't be able to go, then. I guess she still did have some sense of feeling that she wasn't being fair. So we started talking about the idea of a home. She knows people who are in the home who used to be in her church. We're hoping that the experience will be such a positive one that she'll decide to stay permanently rather than staying alone in the house all day.

Evelyn: It is amazing to me to watch the residents at my sister-in-law's nursing home, how they bond with each other and how helpful it is to have one person kind of look after the other. There is one woman, Thelma, who wouldn't be there if her husband hadn't died. She's really quite able, and when she sees me she'll joke and say, "If I slip you ten will you take me home?" And I'll say, "Thelma, I'd love to take you home, but I'd be put in the hoosegow right away. The police would be after me and I wouldn't be worth a plug nickel." But Thelma is always going around holding a hand or rubbing a back and trying to make someone feel better. The bonding that goes on is very interesting. My sister-in-law has a man in the room next to her who thinks she's his wife. Helen will say to me, "I don't understand why he keeps calling me Mickey."

"I think you remind him of somebody," I'll say.

Helen is in his room quite a bit and a lot of her clothes are in his room. When we can't find a piece of her clothing, we look in there, and joke when it's underpants. Of course, the residents do get in bed with each other. It's a warm body. If you have slept with someone all your life and suddenly you are in a bed all by yourself, it's very hard to get used to.

One night, the nurses had a time getting everyone settled in his or her own bed. The gentlemen next door to Helen called out loudly, "It's a fine kettle of fish when you can't go to bed with your own wife!" He was undoubtedly a very dictatorial-type husband.

Every once in a while I have to say, "Mr. Brown, you're upsetting Helen, you really are. Back off just a little bit."

"Why, I've never upset her before in my life!" he'll say.

And I'll say, "Well, you have now." Helen was not treated well in her marriage, her husband was off at sea a lot, and that's the only reason the marriage lasted. So this kind of heavy-handed behavior probably feels normal to her.

Tom: My mother-in-law always has to be going somewhere, even if it's only from this room to that room. What she really wants is to go to Portsmouth, where she was born. She has tried that about a hundred times when she has gotten out of the house in the past. This one particular evening, she got out of her chair by the fireplace. I was across the living room. She suddenly said, "Oh, oh," which means, "I'm falling backwards and I'm going to hit my head on something." It seemed that she invariably aimed for something whenever she fell. She probably fell several hundred times. As she was falling backward, I picked myself up off the sofa, leaped over it, and went into a kind of football-type tackle to get her because her head was aiming for the bricks on the fireplace. I shoved her over to the chair and got her into it. As she flopped down, I was at about the angle of a tackle. I got my hands on the arms of the chair and pushed myself back up. Meanwhile, she looked at me sweetly and said, "Did you hurt yourself?" Racked with pain, I lied through my teeth and said, "No, no." She responded with, "It's a lucky thing I was here to catch you!" She hadn't even remembered falling.

Evelyn: Part of humor is recognizing the component parts of the whole and how they fit together. The humor comes about, as you were saying, when you were bent across on top of your mother-in-law and she looked up at you and made that perfectly incongruous statement. This is the humor in it; that the pieces don't quite fit together the way they should. Because we are looking at small pieces, we find that the blue sky up there is far bluer, far lovelier than it might have been if we hadn't had the negatives to deal with in our lives. We look for the little things, remember the little things, and we cherish the good times. Yesterday was John's birthday and I remember that a year ago I ignored his birthday. He was at day care. But this year, I decided to do something. So I kept telling him it was his birthday all day long, kept singing *Happy Birthday* to him, and we always sing "For he's a jolly good fellow." It was really a lot of fun, reliving the jokes of the past, and I think he enjoyed it—for the moment.

I've got to tell you a story about John. He was not a traveler and I said at one point, if I were ever going to get to Europe it was going to be that year. I knew John wasn't going to want to take a trip. So I just said to him, "Honey, I'm going to France. You can come with me or you can stay at home, whichever, but I'm going." I wish I had done that a long time ago because he decided he would go. So we spent the summer getting passports, buying clothes, getting every book in the world. It was a wonderful trip. I loved every minute of it. We arrived in Paris at six o'clock in the morning, and taking the advice of a lot of people, we did not go to bed, just stayed up. I walked John all over Paris. We went to the d'Orsay Museum and spent three hours there, had lunch, fooled with our money, ordered in French—it was wonderful. That night we had dinner with our tour group. And the next morning in the coffee shop, John was looking around, and said to me, "Where are we?" I didn't know whether to laugh or what. I said to him, "Honey, we're in Paris." If I had said to him, "We are on the moon," he couldn't have been more surprised. He said, "We're in Paris—how did we get to Paris?" The interesting thing is that after that initial question he seemed to catch on to the fact that we weren't home and were in some strange place, and each day he got into the France deal a little bit better. He had a wonderful time, thoroughly enjoyed himself. But to my dying day I will still hear him say, "Where are we?"

Ellen: Does your husband wander at all?

Evelyn: John doesn't have past memory. Many Alzheimer's patients can remember a lot about the past, but he cannot remember anything about the past, really nothing beyond the moment. He hasn't been able to since the symptoms began. The house we've lived in for forty-three years is all he knows; it is his home. So I'm not saying he won't wander but so far it hasn't been one of our problems. But my mother-in-law did wander. An incident occurred with her that shows how something awful can turn around and be something wonderful.

Mother was always trying to go home. I would arrive at her apartment to find this five-foot-two, ninety-pound woman ready to go. She would have had actually taken the mattresses off the beds, rolled and tied them, unscrewed the light bulbs, taken the toilet paper out, emptied the drawers, and was set to go. I would say, "Oh Mother, the movers just called me and they can't come today, they will come tomorrow." And we would have to make the beds again and do all that work. One particular time, she was alone for fifteen minutes. It was pouring rain, around six o'clock in the evening, and she actually left, with two coats on, carrying a box that had just costume jewelry in it. It was not really cold, but it was winter-coat weather, and when John got to the apartment, she was gone. There had been someone with her fifteen minutes before, but just in that short time she took off. The police helped us look. One son stayed at her apartment, I stayed at our house, and John went with the policeman. If it hadn't been for the pouring rain, I doubt if the police would have been quite so helpful. At one o'clock in the morning a taxicab pulled up in front of the apartment. The cab driver had picked Mother up a couple of miles from her apartment and recognized what the problem was. He told her he would take her home and she kept describing where she lived. He would drive to the different apartment complexes and she would say, "No, this isn't it." He kept taking her around until he got her to the right one. It was truly a Good Samaritan story. He would not take one penny more than the money on the meter. He said, "This could have been my mother."

Mother used to also get away from me sometimes in department stores. We'd have lunch in the store and do a little shopping. She was so tiny that I would lose her amid the racks. The sales people in the store got so they knew me and would see me looking all around. Mother thought this was very funny and would do it on purpose. She'd be peeking around to see who was looking for her. People would be coming down on the escalator and would point to where she was hiding.

Tom: A few years after my mother-in-law moved in with us, we were sitting out on the front porch, one day. She looked at me and exclaimed, "Ted, where have you been?" Ted was her husband who died in 1964. So, trying to get some reality into the situation, I said, "I'm not Ted, I'm Tom, your son-in-law."

"I haven't seen you for a while, Ted, where have you been?" she replied.

"I'm not Ted, I'm Tom. Ted died twenty years ago," I repeated.

"You're my husband."

"No, I'm Tom."

"You changed your name."

So I stood up next to her and said, "You see, I'm up here and you're down there, and remember Ted was quite a bit shorter than you are."

So she thought a minute and then said, "So you not only changed your name, you changed your height."

And from there, I went straight to hell in her opinion, because I insisted that I was married to her daughter. She thought that was so terrible that I was married to her and her daughter at the same time!

Evelyn: They lose track of details, but they know they had a husband. John's mother thought that John was her husband and my two sons were her two sons. So that meant I really didn't have a place. When she would introduce me, she would hesitate for a bit. And the first time that this happened, she said, "This is Evelyn, she's uh—(I thought, 'I wonder what she's coming up with') she's my very best friend."

And I was; we were very good friends. But I realized that, to her, John was her husband and my two sons were her two sons. I was outside this constellation.

Jean: That's the way Frances is. She thinks Dick is her husband. After all, it's the right age for their memory. He looks like his father did then. The picture in her bedroom of Dick's father when he was in his forties or fifties looks so much like Dick now. I don't think she knows who I am. I'm the person who cooks the meals. Occasionally, she'll call me Mama. That happens every now and then. But when she says it, she kind of backs off. She realizes it's not right, but she's not sure what is right.

Evelyn: I'm going to tell the story of the diamond ring. John's mother had a very expensive, beautiful diamond ring. She knew how valuable it was, so she would hide it and then not be able to find it. I would get the phone call. "Evelyn, I've put my diamond someplace and I cannot find it. Would you come over and help look for it?" It would be in very strange places, often being hidden somewhere on her person. So we would undress her and search. This particular day, I had gone over around nine o'clock in the morning and by around three o'clock in the afternoon I had looked in every conceivable place in that apartment. Mother was getting agitated and angry with herself. This was in the days of *Mission: Impossible*, if anyone remembers that program, and this took on a kind of "mission impossible" flavor. I was thinking, "I've looked everywhere but I haven't yet looked in the refrigerator." So I went into the refrigerator and started checking the mayonnaise jar, the pickles, etc. Well, lo and behold, there it was in the tub of butter! And I thought, "This is the very last time I'm going to be looking for this ring!" So I said, "Oh Mother, this has got to go to the jewelers to be cleaned after being in that butter." And I thought, "Mission accomplished!" and off it went to the safe-deposit box.

Tom: We had refrigerator problems, too, with my mother-in-law—a totally different kind of problem. We eventually had to wind up installing locks on all the interior doors with dead bolts on the outside, because she was a genius at getting out. We had to get our windows changed so we had quadruple locks on them, or she'd be climbing out the window. It didn't matter that there was an eight-foot drop to the ground. We had caught her trying several times. But, when she first came to live with us, she could roam the house while we slept (or tried to sleep). We found the telephone in the freezer at least three times! That's where it belongs, of course! Believe me, telephones do not like freezers, I can tell you that. Another thing that Alzheimer's patients eventually do, that my mother-in-law was doing around that time, was substituting nouns. They get misplaced, they get substituted, one for the other. She was really upset with me one time because I wouldn't let her go home to her mother and father, who of course had been dead for fifty and sixty years respectively. I told her, "You can't go, you have to stay here tonight, it's raining out, the bus isn't coming (of course there are no buses even near us), it is coming tomorrow. It's not running anymore tonight." She was so frustrated with me, she looked at me and said, "You—you lawyer, you!" And I think what she was trying to say was "You liar, you!"

Once, Clara decided she didn't like being held prisoner in one of the six homes she thought she was living in at that time. She couldn't understand how all six houses had the same decorations. So she said one day, "I'm going to get out of here!" and picked up the phone. All she got was the dial tone, but she said, "Hello, Central—hello, Central!?" I suppose it meant Central Exchange. Who knows how these things pop up—so much out of context. Amazing.

Ellen: Most of those we are referring to here are in-laws, except certainly the spousal relationship between Evelyn and John. I think perhaps, the little bit of distance involved in the in-law relationship provides somewhat of a buffer in dealing with

Alzheimer's patients. The spousal relationship is the most intense, of course, and then the blood relationships.

Jean: In my support group last night, where a lot of people have a parent who has Alzheimer's, several of the folks were saying that every time they forget something they wonder if it's beginning.

Evelyn: One of my sons asked recently, "Mother, I wonder whose genes I have?" Unfortunately, in our family, the incidents of Alzheimer's are astounding. John's mother, her two children, one of her brothers and his two children have been diagnosed. That's six in one family and all were in their sixties.

Ellen: They need you, Evelyn; that's for sure. They need a Pollyanna! You are just amazing; you have such a wonderful attitude. And just think of the joyful gift that you are to your family. What would they do without you? It's hard for you, though.

Evelyn: We don't have a choice with the Alzheimer's, but we have a choice about how we are going to react to it. Every time I see John lose something or not be able to follow along at church where he wants to sing the hymns and tries so hard, I have to stop and think. I can either say, "Oh, isn't that awful?" or I can say, "Aren't I glad I am here to take care of him, aren't I glad he's got what functioning he's got?" I have a choice. Now there are some days when I'm reminded of Charlie Brown who moped around with his head down. I have to say, "Hold your head up, Charlie Brown, and you won't be unhappy." There are days when I am in neutral, I don't go ahead, but I try not to fall back. But essentially we have a choice. We don't have to be doom and gloom, we truly don't. And we only have to do it one day at a time. I have a friend whose husband had viral encephalitis, was paralyzed with the exception of his eyes, and continued to live for twenty-seven years. This lady is such a wonderful woman who has learned so much from her sorrow and pain. We were in high school together and had lost track of each other until our fiftieth reunion and now we are back in touch again. She's the one who said you only have to do it one day at a time. Some days you really only have to do it one hour at a time. That is all you need to do, just get through this one hour or just this one moment. You can make it if you realize that you only need enough strength for this moment. My friend has given me some wonderful tidbits. One of the things she says that I've passed on to so many people is that there are no wrong decisions. There are different decisions. If you make a decision out of love and caring and thoughtfulness, it's not wrong. I've had to rely on that philosophy so many times in dealing with my husband. Even with decisions I've made around the house, I will say to myself, "This decision may not be better, it's just different."

Tom: You don't know how the other decision would have turned out. I work the "Helpline" and if I can get the people on the other end to break out in laughter, then I can begin to talk to them. Usually my mother-in-law has done the same thing the people are telling me their relative is doing and sometimes it was just the night before—something really frustrating. I'll say, "Are you sure you didn't have my mother-in-law over there with you?"

Evelyn: From answering the Helpline, I've discovered that, when there is a dysfunctional family and you add the Alzheimer's person to the picture, it can be a catastrophe. You may have siblings who are at odds and parents who are not getting the proper care while the family fights over whether they should or should not have a certain treatment. The one who should have the most decision-making power is the sibling doing the hands-on care, living at home with the parent. You'll often see cases where there are children living many states away or even outside the country who will say, "There's nothing wrong with Mother." Of course they may only see her for a few minutes a year and don't recognize the onset of dementia. So, the dysfunctional family can be chaotic when Alzheimer's strikes. In Doug Manning's book, *When Love Gets Tough*, he deals with this issue. He says that, often, the child who is left at home, or stays at home to take care of the mother or the father, is the child who is seeking love, acceptance, or approval.

Getting back to funny stories, I have this reputation for getting lost coming out of the garage. I did actually get lost getting out of an underground garage one time. I just kept following the Exit signs and going in what seemed like circles. I eventually had to ask directions to get out of the garage!

My husband and I were driving to Boston a few years ago. When he had his memory he had the reputation of being able to find his way out of Afghanistan in the middle of the night. But at this particular point he was already depending on me to do the navigating. I had the map in my lap, giving him directions. If you have never been to the Boston area you don't know what they do up there. You're on Route 28 and you come to an intersection. There is no sign telling you what to do. It isn't until you've passed the intersection and made your choice that you find out whether or not you've made the right decision. As children, I can remember my mother saying, "Girls, look and see if we're on the right road." Anyway, I didn't make the right decision and we wound up in a section of Boston where, even with the windows shut and the doors locked, I was not sure we were going to get through without someone putting a brick through the window or commandeering the car. It was that scary. And John looked over at me (he has a wonderful sense of humor, truly wonderful; very dry, very low-key) and he said, "Can you tell me where we're going? What have you gotten us into?"

"Well, Honey," I said, "when we get to where we're going we'll be with our son."

It was truly a credit to how much he loves and trusts me, that John just kept driving and didn't say anything. It was also a testimony to how much he wanted to be with his son. Later, when my son heard where we had been he wondered how in the world we got there. The important thing was, I took it literally one minute at a time and we made it!

Ellen: Did you ever hear the story of the two children who were talking about time? The little girl said, "Yesterday is a has-been, it's all gone, never to return, and tomorrow isn't here yet and we have no idea about it at all. But today is a gift." And the little boy said, "Is that why they call it the present?" So I guess the motto is: Live in the moment, be present to the moment and to those around you, and whatever is happening is a gift. That truly is the essence of faith.

Postscript

Some things have changed since Support Group II met. Evelyn reports that John now resides in a nursing home. Still involved with the Alzheimer's Association, Evelyn keeps very busy between her daily visits with John and her volunteer job tutoring dyslexic children. Tom is still covering the Helpline phone at the Alzheimer's Association one day a week. There is more about Tom in the Postscript of "Clara!" (chapter 11). Currently, Jean's mother-in-law is residing in a very nice nursing facility. She has made a good adjustment and, due to receiving a lot of stimulation, is still functioning cognitively at a similar level as before. When Jean leaves some spending money with her, she tells her the money is "too big." She means she wants singles rather than a twenty-dollar bill. When Jean takes her summer clothing to her, she asks how anyone can tell that they are summer clothes. Jean and her family are pleased with the overall care at the facility.

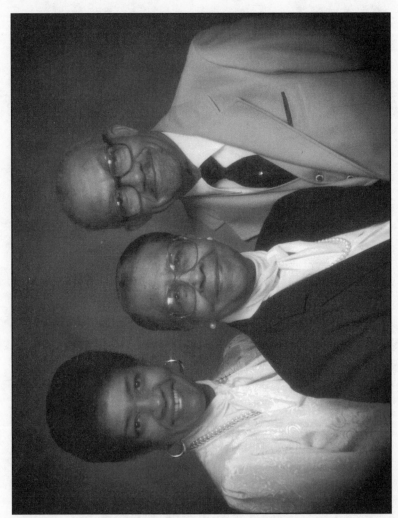

Jean Tucker Mann (at left) with her mother and father

Chapter 6

Random Vignettes

The following kinds of stories can be found and heard everywhere. It is just a matter of looking for them, sometimes even digging for them. This is truly a look at the lighter side of Alzheimer's and an effort to "access mirth."

A caregiver, whose grandmother had recently died, shared wonderfully loving stories with me. It seems her grandmother had the habit of giving the same gifts to her grandchildren every year that they had given her the previous year. Each Christmas, she would put all her gifts away, very carefully. The next year, when she found them again, she believed she had bought them, and subsequently distributed them to her family. They would make bets as to who would get the watch and who would get the sweater or the scarf. One year, this caregiver decided to give her grandmother something that she wouldn't give away. She gave her a fifth of Wild Turkey Bourbon. Her grandmother lived in a small town that practiced temperance almost to a person. The grandmother's son was prominent in the church. He didn't drink, smoke, or curse, and enjoyed being thought of as one of the straight and narrow types. He went to see his mother one night a little before New Year's and thought she had had a stroke. He took her to the hospital and, of course, the doctors found that it was not a stroke, but a major hangover. When the doctors told him that his mother was drunk, he found out who had given her the bottle and was absolutely furious. Everyone in the small town was subsequently to hear that Grandmother was "drunk as a skunk." So much for innovative Christmas presents for people with dementia!

This same wonderful grandmother ran her own business for about fifty years. She would often take her granddaughter on buying trips. Once on a sleeper train, she went to brush her teeth and walked right in the door that said MEN. Her granddaughter was standing in the hall and begged the next man who came along not to go in. When her grandmother emerged and it was pointed out to her that she had been in the men's room, she exclaimed, "Well, it doesn't matter, as long as you get the job done!" Soon after this incident, her son decided she was too old to run her own business and then she started to go downhill fast. One holiday the family was visiting her, and though she seldom talked anymore, she suddenly piped up with a story about having been to the North Pole. She said she had flown there and had made some new friends. She explained that it had been very cold and when asked what she wore, she told them she had a very heavy coat. (This woman lived in the south and had never owned a heavy coat.) She then told them that it was very lonely at the North Pole, that there were not many people, but there were plenty of animals. Each one of the children and grandchildren started to get up and go in the kitchen where they lost it, howling with laughter. They could see how sincerely their grandmother believed that she had made that trip. Proof positive that Alzheimer's patients have new and exciting things happen every day.

Another tale involved a family gathered for a holiday dinner. As they sat down, they realized Grandpa was nowhere in sight. They finally found him in the bedroom. He had every one of his daughter's blouses on, one on top of the other, and he looked very pleased with his accomplishment!

One of the cutest stories I've heard was related to me by a friend regarding her visits to an elderly nun. The nun resides in a nursing home and is pleasantly demented. My friend took her a pair of tennis shoes because she had been having problems with her feet. The nun was so excited when she saw the shoes; she kept touching them and smiling. She had never had a pair of tennis shoes before. Finally, when they were on her feet, she walked down the hall. As they passed the nurses' station, my friend signaled to the nurses and they all made a big fuss over the shoes. When bedtime came, the nun kissed her friend goodnight and then looked fondly over at the shoes and said, "Good night, shoes."

Someone else told me about a day spent with her mother who resides in a nursing home. At lunchtime they were sitting in the dining room with the ladies that were usually at her table. When it came time for dessert, my friend's mother said, "This is very nice, but I'm getting tired of paying for all these lunches every day!" The family recently visited this lady for her eighty-sixth birthday party at the nursing home. One of the relatives gave her a five-dollar bill in a card. She looked at the money in consternation. "Why this isn't very much money." The family asked her why she needed money, as some of them forked over a few more dollar bills. "Tips," she said, "I need it for tips." She also worried about having lost her diamond ring and though the family assured her that it was in a safe-deposit box, she continued to believe she had lost it. When asked why she needed the ring, she replied, "To show everybody I'm not a pauper." When her husband was living, she accused him of sleeping too much. Toward the end of his life, he lost a lot of weight. The woman she shares the room with is mostly bed-confined and is very thin. She often tells her family, "Now just look over there at Dad, he's still doing the same thing, thin as a rail and sleeping all the time." She will often go over and try to shake the poor lady awake, calling her by her husband's name.

◆   ◆   ◆

A man told me the story of an aunt's battle with Alzheimer's. The aunt was well into her seventies when it reached the point that she no longer recognized her family. She had been complaining bitterly about the loss of her clothes, saying someone had stolen them. One day she happened to see herself in a mirror and began a tirade of reprimands, accusing the person in the mirror of having been the thief! Ironically, she recognized the dress but not herself. That is part of the unpredictability with regard to memory in advanced Alzheimer's. You never know what they may or may not remember at any given moment, and they can really catch you off guard.

Doctors are great resources for stories. Some I have worked with have provided me with material for this and the "Hospital Happenings" chapter. One doctor was approached by the house-keeping department of a life-care facility and asked to sign off on allowing a lady to keep her dead parakeet. She wanted to put it in a plastic bag and keep it in her freezer so that she could still get up every morning and pet it. This was actually approved, with the understanding that she would only pet it through the plastic. The woman was still managing marginally in her apartment with the support services of the facility. Proof that love shared with even the smallest of creatures is enriching.

◆   ◆   ◆

Someone I've known since high school lost a beloved aunt to Alzheimer's. She was only in her late sixties at the onset. Before the family was aware of her impairment, they would all go for dinner to the fancy country club to which this aunt belonged. Somehow, people seem more aware of other people's behavior at a country club, particularly when it comes to table manners. It got to the point that the family had to coach the aunt on proper etiquette. One evening, she had had it with their nagging and shouted loudly, "Don't tell me how to act at my club!" That having been said, she proceeded to pick up her soup bowl and loudly slurp down her soup. It wasn't at all funny at the time, needless to say. They were all numb with embarrassment. But looking back, my friend says she has to chuckle when she thinks about it.

A woman I know at the hospital had a lot of stories about her encounters with her mother who is now deceased. The encounters that we talked about indicated that her mother was enjoying herself, at least some of the time. Prior to her husband's death and in the early stages of dementia, this mother would do some of the classic things, such as burning a pot on the stove. She had enough common sense remaining to have agreed with her husband and family that it was time to move into a life-care facility. Realizing that something was happening, and that it was getting to be too much to live alone in a large colonial house, she set about with her husband to do a lot of the work involved in the move. She still had plenty of energy.

After her husband died she went steadily downhill. She fell and broke her hip. Soon after, when her daughter visited, she told her enthusiastically that she had been playing volleyball that afternoon. She also talked about having taken a walk with her husband, now deceased, and said that they had been playing bridge with their friends that very day. Given to wandering, she needed restraints and was kept near the nurses' station in a geri-chair.* The nurses had nicknamed her Houdini because no matter which way they tied the posey restraint,† she would work and work at it until she got it untied. The irony was that they would look over at her, afraid that she would get up on the bad hip and injure it again, and she would be sitting there with a smile on her face, folding the posey and putting it neatly in her lap. She had met the challenge and beaten it! Who cared about wandering at that point? As this special lady progressed in walking with her walker in physical therapy, she amused everyone by calling her new way of walking her "creepy-crawly walk."

Another caregiver told me the story of her mother's descent into Alzheimer's. She said it began with a strange remark that she used all the time: "Oh, this monkey on my back." This would refer to things, such as losing something or everyday little mistakes. She knew she was slipping. The family sat down with her after she was diagnosed and explained what was happening. She unwillingly gave up the keys to her car. The family said they had to keep a sense of humor about what subsequently happened or they would have gone into a severe collective depression. Their mother started to have lots of visions and experiences that were very strange. She was always concerned about the children and other people who were getting into her apartment through a hole in her bedroom closet. Showing their mother that there was really no hole did no good. The children still got in and they were also seen in the trees outside her apartment. She would talk about "the children in the treetops" when she sat on her balcony. Then she began not recognizing her surroundings and sometimes her family. She would call her daughter and say that she knew she

---

*A *geri-chair* is a large, well-padded chair with a tray attached for meals and to keep the patient secure.

†A *posey restraint* is a wraparound vest that can be tied to a chair to keep the patient secure.

was in her apartment but these were not her belongings. When she would knock on their door and insist that THEY were in the wrong apartment, the neighbors above and below patiently directed her to her own apartment. For a period of time she denied knowing one of her daughters, which was very upsetting. That soon passed. Then, her husband became two people and she began setting the table for three. The family deduced that the reason for this might have been that she split the warm, friendly, nice husband and the tired, grouchy, sometimes angry husband in two, thereby having two husbands. They waited for the time when she would refuse to set the table for the angry one, but that didn't happen. Toward the end of her life, this lady resided in a nursing home. In the beginning, she would somehow get a newspaper and be looking up apartments when her family visited. She was all ready to move one day and greeted them with a raincoat over one arm and a lamp in the other. When she finally settled in, she seemed to grow fond of one of the men in the unit and told her family that he always took her out for dinner (he escorted her to the dining room). She was concerned about how these meals were being paid for and the family asked the administrator to tell her how the system worked. She continued to be concerned about how much money this man was spending on her.

This woman's daughter had the good fortune of having a similar experience to my own, in terms of her mother's response to her when she visited. She would make remarks like, "This is just heaven, that you are actually here with me." That is a sign, once again, that the Alzheimer's patient's reality often boils down to "the loving response." There are those who have had the opposite experience—rejection, which is very painful. It may just be a matter of good or bad luck, as to the particular part of the brain that is affected by the plaques and tangles* that cause it to malfunction.

---

*Microscopic senile plaques are found in the memory area of the brains of Alzheimer's patients. They consist of degenerating nerve endings surrounding a protein core (amyloid).

◆ ◆ ◆

A social worker, who visits people in the community, told me about a few of her experiences. She says she marvels at the tenacity of the human spirit. Some of the caregiving spouses of Alzheimer's patients demonstrate great patience and understanding, and are able to manage in the most amazing circumstances. Visiting one such couple, the social worker was greeted by the wife at the door and then saw the patient rapidly approaching her. He seemed quite agitated and said, gesturing toward his wife, "This woman! I don't know what she thinks she's doing. She is always trying to feed me, then she tries to undress me and even take my pants off. I don't know what she wants and she just won't leave me alone!"

Making another home visit, the social worker was talking to the wife at the kitchen table, giving her tips on how to manage her failing husband. Meanwhile, he sat at the table eating his breakfast of oatmeal and coffee. Occasionally, he would be listening to them and the spoonful of oatmeal would go into the coffee cup instead of in his mouth. When he started to drink the coffee a bit later, he looked at his wife and the social worker and with great irritation in his voice said, "Now who did this!?"

There is a kind of phenomenon that occurs with some patients at various points in their descent into the confusion of Alzheimer's. I call it "cloning." My aunt, for instance, cloned my mother. It always seems to be directed at the closest, most beloved relatives, siblings, children, etc. When the family would gather to have dinner with my aunt, there was a period of months that she would get very anxious and continue to ask me, "Where is she?" When this first began, I thought she was talking about some friend who had suddenly popped into her mind. I soon discovered that she would point toward where my mother lived and say, "You know, the girl that lives right around the corner down there." Even though I would point out that mother was there, she would still not be satisfied and continue to say, "I don't understand it, she should be here, too." At that time, my aunt's language skills had faded a lot and her questions were not clear. We could figure out what she meant. Of course, she had another sister who had died thirty years ago, to whom she may have been referring, but my next story makes me tend to think it was more likely the cloning phenomenon.

The following story involves a woman in her eighties proudly showing a friend of mine pictures of her two sons. They were enlarged portraits of them taken recently. This woman was pleasantly demented, with aides staying with her in her apartment round the clock. She suddenly started making references to "the other two," and when asked what she meant, said, "You know my boys, they are outside riding their bikes and I sometimes worry about them." When it was pointed out that her only boys were the ones right there in the picture, all grown up, she replied, "You just don't understand, they are here, and they are fine, but it's the other two I worry about." She only had two sons and she had cloned them—adult sons and child sons. This probably provided some kind of comfort or a sense of continuity for her.

During dinner with a friend, Jean Tucker Mann, recently, she told me of the journey she had shared with her father. The Alzheimer's victim was her mother. In the earlier stages of the memory loss and confusion, the couple celebrated their golden wedding anniversary. Because she could no longer navigate well enough to shop for herself, Jean took her mother out to buy a dress and accessories for the big anniversary celebration to come. On the day of the affair around 9 A.M., Jean received a call from her father. He spoke in a low voice, asking her if she could "talk to Mother." "Is there something special you want me to talk to her about?" "Well," replied Dad, "it is nine o'clock in the morning, the party doesn't begin until 3 P.M., and your mother is completely dressed, hair combed, jewelry on, sitting in a chair in the living room, saying she's just waiting." Jean then understood the problem. Her mother could no longer judge time, in terms of how much there was between 9 A.M. and 3 P.M. She spoke to her on the phone and carefully explained that she should take off her dress and put on a robe, because she had to eat breakfast. She promised she would call her in time to get ready for the party. Her mother was very punctual, so she promised to allow her plenty of time. She wouldn't let her mother be late or have to feel rushed. The mother complied with her daughter's wishes and all went well. She did very well at the party, as most of her social graces were still well intact. It was just that "time thing"!

Another vignette from Jean involved her mother's developing a kind of permanent tight little scowl, with pursed lips. After a few days, Jean happened to be at the house when her father was hanging out the laundry. Her mother had never had a dryer. She had always insisted on hanging her wash outside in the fresh air. As her mother went to the window and saw what was happening, she got an even greater look of consternation on her face. Jean begged her mother to tell her what was wrong. She finally was able to get it out, because by this time, her speech was fading fast. "That's MY job!" she said. Jean tried her best to explain that Dad wasn't taking over her mother's jobs to take them away from her, but that he just wanted to give her a rest and have her take it easy for a while. But the mother wasn't happy about any of it. She had always been a perfect "domestic engineer" and resented having her work usurped by her husband, or anyone else, for that matter.

◆   ◆   ◆

An admissions coordinator of a local nursing home was giving a tour to some folks. They went into an empty room and the family looked everything over carefully, including checking out the bathroom. Imagine their surprise when they opened the bathroom door to discover someone sitting on the "throne," completely unruffled, as if these encounters occurred every day. They did! This patient's room was down the hall and she wandered a lot. It was not unusual for her to be found in any one of the bathrooms on the unit. This nursing home had also recently admitted a man who was a pacer. The staff knew the way to handle that problem. Anytime they had an errand to do or had to go off the floor for some reason they just took Sam with them. It kept him slender and happy!

A co-worker told me about some of the antics her grandmother liked to pull. Grandma would do some of her own self-care, such as bathing. But it was getting tricky because she'd miss a lot of important places. So her daughter would sit her down on the covered toilet seat and give her a sudsy washrag. Grandma had been a nurse and her daughter was not shy about stripping down and taking a bath in front of her. So she proceeded to stand in front of the sink and wash herself to encourage Grandma to do the same. Without missing a beat, Grandma came out with, "What you see when you don't have a gun!" She just kept right on washing.

This same wonderful grandmother had the ability to remember who her son-in-law was even when she didn't know the rest of her family. "He's a great guy," she would say. She sometimes wouldn't recognize her own daughter but it would still be "Kevin, this" and "Kevin, that," always in complimentary terms. One day her daughter asked her what she was going to do if she, her daughter, should die and not be around to take care of her any more. Again, without missing a beat, she said, "Marry Kevin."

Another day, this same witty lady was with her daughter and

son-in-law and they were getting ready to take her out. She looked at Kevin and said, "Isn't he wonderful."

"Yes, he certainly is," Helene responded.

"Mother, do you know who I am?"

"I'm your daughter," she replied.

"No," said Helene, "I am YOUR daughter."

"No you're not," replied the mother. "My daughter is better looking than you are." This grandmother missed her calling as a stand-up comedian!

At a local nursing home, two stories recently were related to me. It was Saturday afternoon, and the entertainment for the day was in progress. When the singer finished singing Whitney Houston's *I Will Always Love You*, she made the remark, "Isn't that a great song?" One of the residents piped up with, "Yeah, too bad you destroyed it!"

On a different day they were doing gross motor exercises* with the dementia day-program group. The movement was to pretend to be pulling on a parachute, hands going up and then pulling down. The leader said, "You know, folks, a parachute, looks like a big sheet." Someone in the group said something that sounded like, "Per cow?" The leader happened to live on a farm and actually had cows, so her response was, "No, cows sleep on straw, they don't get sheets." Someone else said, "No, she said, 'Percale' (a brand of sheets)." She was just pronouncing it as if it had no "e" at the end!

I met with the director of an adult daycare program in a local nursing home. What a wealth of material she had to contribute!

---

*Exercising arms and legs as opposed to fingers.

She started by telling me that one day she found one of the day-care patients in her office, tearing out the pages of her day-timer calendar book. Other objects in her office had been moved or disappeared from time to time, but none had the impact of the loss of the pages of the day-timer. The office was unusual, in that it didn't really have four walls; so the access was easy.

Another daycare participant was very focused on holidays, which had been the highlight of her life. When Easter came, she told the other folks that it was Christmas and she had many things to do. She had her cards to write and gifts to buy and wrap. Someone in the group piped up loudly with, "Well, just how many Christmases are there?"

Someone else in the group was a wanderer. Her daughter, who was a teacher, would drop her off in the morning before going to school. One particular morning they observed some wildlife in the back wooded area. Occasionally a fox or a deer could be seen. Later in the day when she was waiting for her daughter to pick her up one of the staff members started to walk out the door and she shouted, "Don't go out there! There are bears out there!" In her mind, whatever she had seen—fox, deer—had grown into a bear. The staff joked about using "the bears" as a way to prevent her from wandering off the unit, but of course, they didn't.

There was a woman in the group who liked to hoard things. The staff would find up to twenty packets of sweetener in her socks or underclothing.

One of the men must have been a frustrated waiter, though he had never really worked as one. He loved to help and prided him-self on his skill at serving and clearing. The problem was he would clear the food away right after serving it, thereby not giving people a chance to eat. This would usually take place at snack time when the staff would allow him to assist. His wife said he did the same thing at home when they had guests. There was absolutely no time built in to his routine for consuming whatever he was serving. It was immediately whisked away. The staff allowed him to pour juices but they no longer let him pour coffee because he had been known to take the pot out of the machine while it was still dripping. He put an apron on, a towel over his arm, and occasionally sang "Happy Birthday" to the others, even when there was no birthday!

While at a lacrosse game with her family, one woman's daughter-in-law happened to notice that people around them were looking and laughing. Mom had taken off her sweater and was sitting there in her bra. She felt warm and it was the natural thing to do—so she did!

Disrobing is a common problem with dementia. The day program has had several incidents of various pieces of clothing being removed. They try to quickly whisk the patient into the office. Sometimes they are faced with the challenge of finding the pieces of clothing that have been removed. At times a bath towel is put around the person as he or she is taken into the room to reclothe.

The art therapist was running a class in which the folks were fabricating things out of tinfoil. She tried to get the group's creative juices flowing by suggesting that one of the items looked like an airplane. One participant heard this, looked at his watch, and said, "I've got to meet Johnson at the airport!" He became insistent that he must leave so they took him to a phone in the office and then fabricated a call to the airport. "Hello, Johnson, we are wondering what time to meet you at the airport. Oh, not until 8 P.M. Okay, we'll be there." They calmed the man down by explaining that they would have to leave in about four hours. He was fine, went home with his family at the end of the day, and never mentioned it again.

Another man, we'll call him Bill, had lived in a high rise, and though the daycare program was in a three-story building, he always insisted that he wanted to go to the seventh floor. To distract him from his concern about always being on the wrong floor, they linked him up at the table with another gentlemen, Tom, with whom they felt he would get along. Tom got up rather rapidly and went to a recliner, which was his habit after lunch. Bill immediately tried to leave the room to wander, so they took him over to Tom, saying, "Don't you two want to spend some time talking?" Bill bellowed to Tom, "You left me alone at the lunch table!" The coordinator suggested that perhaps Tom had just wanted to get to the recliners quickly in order to save the other one for Bill. Bill then said, "No, he didn't, he wanted to save the other one for you." The coordinator said, "No, Bill, I'm a married woman." Bill asked how long she had been married and she said eight years. He responded with, "Boy, have you got a lot to learn!"

A man in the group was very fastidious about cleanliness. He was found one day in the bathroom, washing out his "disposable bladder-control undergarment." Much to his wife's dismay, she said he did this quite frequently at home also. He would hang them neatly over the shower curtain. One day, this same man proudly told the rest of the group that he was going out to dinner at the Belvedere. He claimed he was going with a twenty-one-year-old. Later it was revealed that he was going out with twenty-one members of his church group. A little wishful thinking, maybe!

One day, the center was doing a fancy luncheon for the group, just to keep up their social graces. One participant who was very impaired and rarely said anything coherent piped up, "We ought to have grace." One of the others chimed in with, "Praise the Lord."

A small group had been taken to the city fair. A call came back to the center saying they had lost Daniel and Millie. Everyone was on the bus when it was realized that they were missing. Staff members scanned the grounds where the two had been and finally found them standing in line for the Ferris wheel, holding hands.

On another occasion, a client was coming to the center for the first time. He was very angry about being there. The group leaders were greeting him and offering him a bun and cup of coffee, when he shouted out, "Shove it!" One of the others retorted with, "Where?" Everyone burst out laughing and from then on the group leaders found that humor was a good way to deal with this partic-ular person. He responded to joking and laughter.

One day, the bus was taking the clients home and a woman refused to get off at her stop because she didn't recognize her house. After some coaxing, she finally got off the bus and went to her family member. Once in the house, she agreed that it was her home. That particular day, the outside of the house had been deleted from her memory.

Reportedly, every now and then there is a day when it seems a kind of "sleeping sickness" takes over the group and they all seem lethargic and sleepy, as though it is contagious. One particular day two individuals were seated in the group, leaning toward one another with their heads touching. It was so cute, the leader took a photo. They were actually asleep, holding each other up!

A staff member once noticed that a woman was holding a pair of dentures. She was smiling broadly, clearly showing that they were obviously not hers. The staff members had to go around and ask everyone to smile for them in order to find out to whom the dentures belonged. They found the owner, who had just casually taken them out and left them on the table.

A client at another center was found in the bathroom washing her dentures in the toilet. Luckily they found her in time and got them thoroughly scrubbed with soap and hot water before she resumed wearing them!

One gentleman had a mustache that had turned gray. He used his wife's mascara to darken it to give him a more youthful appearance. One day he came to the center with a blue mustache. He had used his wife's eye shadow by mistake.

A woman in the group was asked what her name was. She responded, "I'm me." When asked where she was, she said, "I'm right here." When asked what time it was, "It's now."

During one daycare session of sensory stimulation the discus-sion centered on the water and the beach. The group was asked to think about what their memories were of the beach. One man piped up with, "Under the boardwalk!" Everyone burst out laughing. They never got the rest of the story, just made their own assumptions.

Another nearby nursing home has a DDP (Dementia Day Program). One day one of the attendees asked what DDP stood for. The leader told her. She thought a minute and then said, "Hmm, I took Latin and I know 'mentia' means mind and 'de' means down. So, if I'm here it must mean I'm losing my mind."

The leader was telling a story about something involving "a one-horse open shay." She explained "shay," saying it was an open carriage. One woman piped up with, "I know how to spell it, it's not 's-h-a-y,' it's 'c-h-e-z.' "

A woman I know through church shared some stories about her aunt who is now in her late seventies and suffers from Alzheimer's. She and her husband live with their daughter and granddaughter. One evening the family was sitting in the window when the aunt suddenly said, "What a crazy hat that lady has on." Everyone looked around to see what she could mean. There was a tall lamp with a large, ornate lampshade in the corner of the room and she was looking right at it. Mystery solved!

This same aunt has been married to her husband for over fifty years. One night, recently, she kept her husband awake all night by constantly pushing him or poking him, saying, "Move over and make room for Millicent, for heaven's sake!" Millicent is her sister, who, for whatever reason, she believed was a third person in the bed that night.

A woman who lives in a life-care facility* recently told me of an incident that occurred at a gathering that was held there. At one point, one woman said, "Someone came to see me last night." And before she could get another word out, another woman asked, "Was it me?"

The wife of a man who resides in the same nursing home as my mother told me she had taken her husband out for a ride one day. Upon their return he kept telling her he didn't want to go back there, that he wanted to go home. She kept reassuring him but insisted that he had to go back. When asked why, she said, "Because of the Alzheimer's."

"That's okay for them," he said, "but I want to go home!"

A relative of someone else in the same nursing home had a rather hair-raising experience. When her husband was still at home, but sinking into severe dementia, he would go to bed every night at about eight. She would go up at eleven and just after she fell asleep, he would get up and wander. He had a habit of calling the police, and one night his wife woke up, startled, to see a policeman standing over her bed. The policeman said, "Your husband says that you are keeping him prisoner here." Nursing-home placement occurred soon after that incident.

The following story involves a woman in her early eighties who had been impaired by Alzheimer's for about fifteen years. Though severely impaired cognitively, she could still walk and willingly followed directions, which usually involved taking her by the hand and showing her what to do or where they wanted her to go. The main thing was she was pleasant and didn't have catastrophic reactions.†

---

*A *life-care* facility is a place that takes people into apartments when they are well and then moves them into domiciliary rooms or the infirmary as needed, during the remainder of their lives.

†A pronounced, dramatic—usually negative—reaction to some situation or event.

The daughter took this lady to the hairdresser on a regular basis. When she entered the room with all the mirrors, her face lighted up and she walked over and put her hands against her own hands on the mirror. "Hello, it's good to see you," she would say, as if she were meeting a good friend. She no longer knew who her family members were, specifically, but she knew their faces. Obviously, she still knew her own face, but she didn't know it belonged to her. This little scene was played out every time they went to the hairdresser. This family refers to their own journey with their pleasantly demented mother as a "success story." Their philosophy is, it could be so much worse. She is pleasant, she isn't in any pain, and she doesn't seem to be suffering at all.

So once again we see, that though Alzheimer's is an emotionally painful experience for everyone involved, there can be silver linings here and there. If nothing else, there are random moments of mirth to be savored. There are also lessons to be learned. We clearly see in these little stories that patients who have been diagnosed with dementia are living in their own reality and it is different from ours. It is never wise to try to get these folks to "see it our way." Better to go along, try to divert their attention to something else, and then hope that the memory loss comes to the aid of the situation.

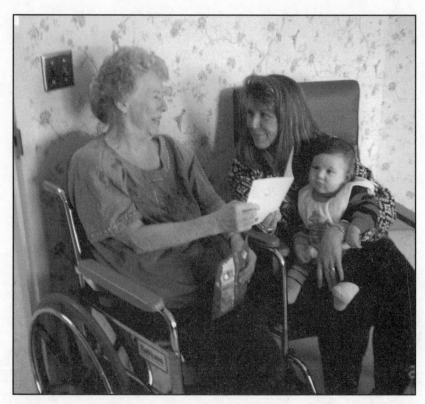
From left: Mary, Maureen, and Kevin

Chapter 7

A Silver-Lining Story

I visited Maureen in her home one evening to interview her for this chapter. Her nine-month-old baby, Kevin, was just finishing his bottle and enjoying cuddling with Mommy. Her husband, David, and their springer spaniel had gone out for a while, as it was felt the dog might disrupt our interview. Kevin, however, was an angel, falling asleep for part of it and being as good as gold during the time that he was awake. A most adorable baby.

Maureen began her story. It is the story of harrowing experiences resulting from a rapid onset of Alzheimer's disease in 1989. Mary, Maureen's mother, had just retired from nursing. During the previous year, she had also overseen the care of her own mother, Maureen's grandmother, who was ill and dying. Mary had been a nurse for thirty years in a hospital in Cumberland, Maryland, where the family had always lived. She was sixty-two and spent her first year of retirement adjusting to her mother's death. She and her husband, Jim, cleaned out her mother's home and sold it.

The first time anything strange was noticed was in 1990 or 1991. Maureen's sister, Marianne, had the folks visiting her in Mississippi. She reported to Maureen that Mother was "acting strange." There wasn't really anything they could put their finger on, just little things. But from then on, all three—Dad, Maureen, and her sister—sensed that something was wrong with Mom. At first they attributed it to the possibility that there had been too much sudden change for her, i.e., retirement and the subsequent loss of her mother.

In this same time frame, Maureen remembers attending a reunion with friends from grade school. One of them worked with Alzheimer's patients. Maureen remembers thinking, "I wonder if it could possibly be Alzheimer's." But then she would quickly put the idea out of her mind. The family was in deep denial regarding this possibility.

By 1992 the family continued to be perplexed. Mary would have periods of acting strangely but then would have equal periods of seeming fine. She and Jim went to Florida annually to visit friends and attend baseball spring training. They usually stayed about a month. The return trip to Cumberland in 1992 was a problem. Mary and Jim were about sixty-six years old at the time. They were as far as Georgia when Mary had a panic attack and couldn't drive. Jim had never gotten his license so could not be of help at that point. He thought Mary was just tired, so they stopped for a couple of nights. They finally had to call their friends in Pompano Beach. The couple drove up to Georgia and, using both cars, drove Mary and Jim back to Cumberland.

Indeed, this could have been a "call to awakening," but it wasn't. After all, Mary had always been sharp and in excellent health all her life. The family thought there must be an explanation for the little problems she was having. Her first visit to the doctor resulted in a diagnosis of the flu. Dizzy spells that followed were attributed to an inner-ear infection. This was believed to be the cause of her problems with balance and memory.

In May of 1992, Mary called Maureen to report that someone had stolen her wallet. She claimed that someone had come right into the house and stolen it. The crime rate was comparatively low in Cumberland and someone entering the house and stealing just the wallet sounded unbelievable. Maureen knew her parents didn't make a habit of leaving the doors unlocked. But her mother sounded very anxious, saying she didn't know what to do, how to report it, or how to replace her credit cards and license. Maureen felt something was wrong because she knew her mother was an intelligent woman who would normally have had no difficulty figuring out what to do in this kind of situation—but now she had no clue. Later Jim found the wallet; Mary had hidden it and then completely forgotten. Nevertheless, denial continued to prevail in the family.

The following Christmas things took a turn for the worse. Mary and Jim drove from Cumberland to Baltimore to be with Maureen and David. On Christmas day Mary was definitely not herself. She didn't want to go to church services. Everyone thought that was really odd but still of no real concern. The previous year had been like a roller coaster and there was still no consistency in the strange behavior. She didn't have an appetite and showed no interest in chocolate, though all the family members were "chocoholics." She expressed a need to go back home. The family once again attributed this behavior to the flu or some unknown physical ailment. A return visit to the doctor resulted in a referral to a neurologist. This time the diagnosis was a carotid artery problem, which was causing a blockage of blood flow to the brain. It was blamed for the memory lapses, panic attacks, and dizziness. Everyone felt relieved. There was a name for it, it had been diagnosed and could be fixed.

By February of 1993 the family had agreed that a workup at Johns Hopkins Hospital was in order. The Cumberland doctor was no longer convinced that the problem was related to blood flow to the brain. Further tests had not borne this out and surgery was not done. It was very difficult for the doctor, who had known Mary and worked with her for many years, to face the fact that it was Alzheimer's. Upon arrival at Hopkins, one of the first things that was done was the mini-mental status test.* Mary did poorly. She and Jim stayed with Maureen from February until May while all the tests were done. The doctors ruled out everything but Alzheimer's. The family was devastated.

From February to July of 1993 the bizarre behavior prevailed. It rocked the family to its very foundation. Back in Cumberland, Mary would have bouts of not recognizing her husband. She would suddenly think he was an impostor, a stranger, and would demand that he leave the house. At times, she became agitated enough to call the police, screaming that there was a man in her home. Cumberland is a small town and what was happening was soon recognized by the neighbors and the police. Neighbors whom Mary had always trusted invited Jim to come to their home any time there was a problem. Later they would walk back with him and invariably Mary would greet him with, "Where have you been? There was a strange man here!" These behavior patterns were clearly very hard on Jim. He never knew when it was going to strike. He and Mary could be sitting at the table having a normal conversation over a cup of coffee and suddenly she would look at him and say, "Where's Jim?"

"I'm Jim."

She'd then go into a tirade, yelling, "No you're not!"

Jim would leave the house, hoping she would calm down if she were left alone awhile. At first he would just stand around the side of the house awhile so he could make sure she was okay. Then he would start going to the neighbor's house and calling her. Again she would tell him of the stranger who had been in the house and how frightened she had been. When Maureen heard these stories, she thought it sounded too bizarre, but then it started happening to her.

---

*A short verbal test given to rule dementia in or out.

Mary went through periods where she thought her mother was alive. Alzheimer's patients often forget what they look like and since Mary looked a lot like her mother, at times she thought it was her mother she was seeing when she looked in the mirror. At one point she even accused Jim of murdering her mother. She tried to call the police, saying, "You killed her, you killed her!"

Jim was devastated. At that point he called Maureen and asked her to come right away, saying he couldn't take it anymore. By the time Maureen arrived her mother was fine. Even Jim said it was like old times. They spent a normal day doing what they had always done. Things were still normal at bedtime that night, but by the next morning it struck. Maureen went out in the hall and her mother passed her with an expression on her face that indicated there was absolutely no recognition. She replied to Maureen's "Good morning" in an obvious effort to fake it. Maureen thought it best to be normal and got breakfast going. Mary asked her daughter how she had gotten to Cumberland. She responded that she had driven. Mary asked what car she had brought and when told, looked out the window and got very upset. She turned to Maureen and said loudly, "That's not your car, that's my daughter's car. I knew you were an impostor!" She became very agitated. Up to that point she had been pleasant, not letting on that she didn't know her daughter, but the car proved to her what she had suspected.

The level of anger that her mother reached frightened Maureen so much that she ran upstairs and called home for her husband to come quickly. The rage was so intense that she feared her mother might come after her with a butcher knife. Instead, she just came up, grabbed her, and told her to get out of the house. The neighbors had given her father a key to their house and he now gave it to Maureen and told her to go there and call for help. Maureen called the doctor and the hospital. This was not considered a reason for hospitalization, as Mary had not harmed anyone. Because their own doctor was away, Maureen got in touch with a doctor whose father had Alzheimer's. He was very empathetic. He told them to bring Mary to the hospital, that he could admit her for adjustment of medications. Maureen called her parents' best friends and they quickly appeared. She then called the house. Her mother answered and seemed fine, acting as though she didn't even know her daughter had been there. Maureen said she had just gotten into town and Mary told her to come right over, that she was looking forward to seeing her. When she walked back to her parents' house, her mother acted as if nothing had happened. She was delighted to see her. This was an hour after she had literally thrown Maureen out, believing she was an impostor.

In order to get Mary to go with them to the hospital, they called a friend who worked there, creating the ruse that she wanted to see Maureen while she was in town. They all drove to the hospital. Admission went smoothly as the friend gently explained to Mary that she felt she should stay a couple of days for a checkup. Mary was very cooperative. They kept her for two days. She seemed fine, enjoying the visits of some of the people with whom she had worked. The family feared the doctors would think they were crazy, but the doctor who was going through something quite similar with his father understood the situation very well. He told them that Mary's calm reaction was normal. She had a sense of security because she was in a familiar place and knew many of the people.

By the second night they had to put a sitter in with Mary because she was trying to leave. The level of her impairment was becoming more obvious as she began "sundowning," a condition that involves the declining of mental status toward evening. After the two days and an attempt to adjust her medications, Mary was released from the hospital. She became a zombie from all the medicines she was taking and Jim was upset about that. He refused to get someone to come in to help with Mary's care. The sitter the family had used for the grandmother came once and Mary physically threw her out. Jim was still at the point where he was embarrassed and didn't want people to see his wife that way. He felt it was better if he just tried to handle her himself.

Maureen recalls telling her friends that she was afraid her father was going to have a stroke from the constant stress. At this juncture, the family really didn't know where to turn. They tried to persuade Mary to go to an adult daycare program but she fought the idea to such a degree that they gave up. Word travels, and no sitter would risk taking the job. Jim finally said he felt the family would have to face the painful fact that a nursing home was the only answer. Mary's closest childhood friend fought this decision, saying "over my dead body will you place Mary in a nursing home." The friend and her husband had a cottage at Deep Creek Lake where the families had spent many summers together. They took Mary and Jim there for a weekend and by early the first day, the friend admitted to Jim that Mary needed to be in a nursing home. She had observed the out-of-control behavior, the agitation, and the constant motion. By this time Jim had lost over twenty pounds, just trying to keep up with her. He wasn't sleeping, he didn't have time to eat, and Mary kept throwing him out of the house.

Maureen remembers how awful it was to be terrified of her own mother. She never knew when Mom would snap. One week when Mary and Jim were visiting in Baltimore for the weekend, Maureen was trying to work on typing her graduate-work papers. At one point Mary came into the room and asked, "Maureen, where is your father?" Maureen knew her father was sitting right in the living room, from where her mother had just come. This was usually the signal that "it" was starting. At first, when these episodes would occur, Jim would take out some kind of identification in hopes of convincing Mary that he was Jim. It never worked.

The Hopkins doctors were perplexed about the rate at which Mary was deteriorating. They admitted to only having seen about six cases where the patients had passed through the various stages so quickly—the bizarre acting-out behavior, wrapping things up and hiding them, believing there were vagrants in the house, not believing it was her house. She constantly would get out a suitcase and start packing, saying they would have to move.

Maureen, her sister, and her father finally had to agree with the doctors that nursing-home placement was their only option. This was in June of 1993. The family ran into problems with the placement because there was no medical reason for hospitalization. There was a brand-new nursing home in Cumberland run by a woman with whom Mary had worked at one time. An opening was anxiously awaited. They happened to all be together when the call came that there was a bed available.

Then the ordeal began. At that point Mary recognized her husband and daughters only some of the time. She was still able to do some things normally. The family asked the doctor to assist them in telling her about the nursing home. He was not very effective in this attempt, probably because he was troubled by it, since he had worked with Mary over the years of her nursing career. The family felt they were "leading the lamb to slaughter." Mary sat there, innocent of all that was going on around her. The suitcase was packed and the family had to deal with their own realization that Mom would never be back in that house again. They told her that she needed to go out to Devlin Manor for a little vacation, but her response was negative. She kept saying, "No, No, I don't want to go . . . don't make me go . . . please don't make me go . . . I'll be good." They explained that Dad needed a little time off and she said, "I won't do anything to Dad." It was all a nightmare. They finally got her in the car. Once at the facility Mary recognized a lot of her former co-workers and was fairly compliant during the admission process. Maureen described herself, her sister, and her father as a pathetic group at that point. They didn't know what was the best thing to do, so they stayed with Mom the rest of the day. They were too miserable to do anything but pace. Mary kept asking questions and saying she wanted to go home. The only way they could keep her calm was to say it was only for one night.

The family finally left, but when they returned the next day, the first thing Mary said was, "I'm ready to go now." Maureen suggested that they all stay awhile and walk around. They walked and they walked. Mary kept saying, "Let's go—go," and they all thought she meant let's get out of this place. Then she would remark on how beautiful the scenery was, as the mountains were visible. Finally, Mary exclaimed, "Would you believe it, all the money we pay for this motel room and we can't even go outside and enjoy the beautiful scenery!"

Later in the day, Mary sat down and was suddenly fully aware of where she was. She began to berate her family. "What have you done to me?" They replied that it would all be okay, but she was having none of it. "I know where I am, I'm at Devlin Manor. How could you do this to me? My own family—you traitors!" She began to cry. The family was devastated. Jim approached her and she pushed him away. The only one she would let near her was Maureen, whom she said was "the only innocent one" (though no one could figure out why she said that). Maureen walked with her. Mary's father had been in a nursing home for ten years and when he died her mother made her promise never to place her in one. She never did. So, when Mary had a lucid moment and realized what was happening, she felt betrayed. She cried for quite a while and said she would die there. Then it was over. It was time for medicines and she was distracted. From that day on she never again mentioned where she was or seemed aware of it. Most of the time she thought she was back at work. In fact, prior to her retirement, she had actually hired some of the people who now worked at the nursing home and had been their supervisor at the hospital. It was similar enough to a hospital setting for her to feel somewhat at home.

A couple of weeks later when Maureen came for a visit she saw her mother sitting behind the nurses' station desk. Someone had given her a ledger and she was busily writing figures in it. She had her glasses on and looked happy. When Mary looked up, Maureen said, "Mother, I'm really sorry to bother you at work but I just stopped by to say hello."

Mary continued to do well under the guise of being a nurse employee. She helped straighten the linens and one day while passing the nurses' station she yelled at the aides for being too noisy. The administrator related this story to Maureen and added, "You know, your mom was right, too." One of the aides said later, "You can tell Mary used to be a supervisor, because she'll start telling me what to do and I'll start to do it. Then I remember that she is a patient. But she really knows what needs to be done." Mary also helped out by pushing people in their wheelchairs up and down the halls.

Within a couple of months, during the fall of 1993, all the activity gradually faded. Mary's awareness declined and she didn't think she was at work anymore. She became aware of very little, and sadly, reached the point where she didn't recognize her husband and daughters. Her ability to speak faded and much of what came out was garbled. After three or four words, her sentences would deteriorate into gibberish. She still knew people sporadically, but by Christmas 1993, when people visited, she knew very few.

Just as Maureen had feared, two days after Mary had gone into the nursing home, Jim had a stroke. It was fairly severe, affecting his left side, but fortunately not affecting his memory or speech. The speech was slightly slurred at first, but is clear now. He still has some difficulty walking and doesn't have much use of one arm but is able to manage living at home alone. His friends and neighbors do his grocery shopping and take him to the bank.

From the time Jim had the stroke in July of 1993 until that Thanksgiving he did not visit Mary. He had been in the hospital and rehab for three months. After that, he was afraid it would upset her to see him walking with a walker or even a cane. Now he visits Mary two or three times a week, but it took him a long time to feel comfortable doing it. During visits he would be so painfully aware of both of their impairments that it upset him to the point of tears. Maureen said it was a sweet scene though, because Mary would put her hand up to Jim's face and mutter something that indicated she didn't want him to cry.

At the time of this writing, Mary doesn't really recognize anyone, but she is glad to see her family when they visit. It is as if she sees familiar faces and that gives her pleasant feelings. She will occasionally say the name "Jim," but she can't have a conversation with him. She doesn't appear to understand much of what is said to her, but if asked how she feels, sometimes she answers, "Okay." She will parrot what others say. "Oh Mom, I love you" comes back, "I love you."

Concurrently, at that particular point in time, there was something "developing" between Maureen and David. They had been married for eighteen years. The first few years they didn't think much about children, as both were busy finishing their degrees. David had to take a medication for colitis, which had a side effect of lowering his sperm count. After about ten years of marriage they were checked out and it was discovered that they were not conceiving because of the medication. He could not go off it so they made peace with the fact that a baby might not be in the picture. They felt if they did conceive it would be fine and if they didn't that would be all right, too. Maureen was about forty and David was soon to be fifty. David was eventually taken off the medication, but the doctor told them not to bet on the possibility of a pregnancy. Having given up, they weren't even thinking about it. They got a dog and figured they could lead a full life without children.

Maureen decided to have a surprise birthday party for David. She told a friend she hadn't gotten him a present yet and was told a story of someone who had told her husband she was pregnant for his fiftieth birthday gift. Little did Maureen know, but at the time of the party, she was actually pregnant. About a month later David got his surprise gift when it was confirmed. This all occurred about eight months after the harrowing events surrounding the Alzheimer's diagnosis. Kevin was born in June of 1994.

Before he was born, Maureen visited her mother. During the whole nine months of pregnancy Mary had not noticed and had said nothing. Upon seeing her daughter's nearly nine-month belly, however, she suddenly asked, "Are you pregnant?" Maureen replied happily that she was. After the baby was born, when Maureen was rocking him in her arms because he was crying, Mary said, "Give him to me." Another time when he was crying, she said, "Oh, my darling, what's wrong?" During one recent visit when Kevin was seven months or so, she reached out to help feed him by leaning over and helping Maureen hold the bottle.

The irony in this whole story involves the timing of Kevin's birth. At the writing of this chapter he is ten months old. As the only grandchild, the family dubbed him their "Alzheimer's gift baby." Kevin's birth is a true "silver-lining" story. It lifted the whole family up and gave them new life and new hope.

Maureen recalls her lifelong relationship with her mother, saying there were the normal little problems that are in all parent/child relationships, but that basically it had been an excellent one. Her mother was her biggest supporter, always telling her she was proud of her and lauding her accomplishments. As most mothers, she listened with great interest to everything her children told her about themselves. Maureen and her mom would have lunch together, watch old movies, cry, and eat chocolate together.

While the family was going through the traumatic times leading up to the Alzheimer's diagnosis and even thereafter, there was no time to really think about the loss they were experiencing. Even at the time that Mary was being diagnosed, Maureen thought it wouldn't actually happen for a couple of years.

She felt there would be plenty of time for reflection and dealing with all of it later. Little did any of them know that within five months Mary would basically be totally gone from them. Maureen said her mother was her rock and the realization of the depth of the loss, when it hit, was monumental. She felt orphaned and abandoned. Then she became pregnant with Kevin and a new life cycle began. She was losing her mother, but here was a child to whom she could give all her love, attention, and affection.

Jim felt his life was over. Between the stroke and the guilt he felt for placing Mary in a nursing home, he was bereft. He knew, intellectually, there had been no other choice, but had to work through his feelings while struggling with recovering from the stroke. Kevin is his first and only grandchild. It has given him such a new lease on life to be a grandfather. Maureen wonders if her father could have even gone on if Kevin hadn't come along. Mary had been his rock. She had been a super wife and super mom. The whole family feels they would never have recovered from the blow of this cruel loss if it weren't for Kevin. As a life so central to this family's well-being was ebbing away, it seemed as if a new precious life was being given as a gift of compensation.

Maureen goes to Cumberland to visit her mother about once a month. She says she's really in trouble if she doesn't have Kevin with her because everyone looks forward to seeing him. Even though Mary has no idea who Maureen is or who Kevin is, she lights up every time she sees them and continues to be able to form phrases or sentences about Kevin. Maureen remembers that one of the only arguments she ever had with her mother was about why she didn't have children. She wanted grandchildren so badly and Maureen feels it is unfair that she isn't able to be well and really enjoy the child. However, the family is grateful for the fact that it appears that she really does enjoy seeing Kevin and still is able to say words about him. They feel that the words are a kind of sign that she does somehow know. Mary will rub the baby's cheek or pat his head and say, "Oh, darling, oh, my darling." She appears to really enjoy him. The family wants Kevin and his grandmother to be a part of each other's life for as long as possible. At this point, Mary has reached a kind of plateau. Maureen knows she will get worse, but no one really knows what the future will bring.

Mary is physically well and can walk. Last year, however, she fell and sustained a hairline fracture of the hip. Surgery wasn't needed, but she didn't walk for months and everyone was afraid she would lose her ability mainly by forgetting. She was in a wheelchair for a while, but with therapy and a lot of time, she learned to walk again. However, she spends most of her time in her room sitting in a chair. She has a very nice roommate, who is in the nursing home for physical reasons but is very alert mentally. The roommate's family lives in town and they visit her every day. They like Mary and always include her in their visit, even though she doesn't communicate with them. Hence, Mary gets a good deal of daily attention and stimulation.

Maureen brought out some pictures of Mary, older ones and ones taken recently. She looks well and happy. The nurses love her. They fix her hair and lightly make up her face. Maureen says, "Whatever little world Mom is in, she is very pleasant, the staff loves her, and she is happy." There is a man at the nursing home whose wife is a patient, who tells Maureen that she is lucky because her mother is so pleasant. His wife is always agitated and difficult to handle. So from that standpoint, not only is this a "silver-lining story," because of Kevin, it is also a kind of "success story." At this point along the way, the term "success story" is, of course, only relative. Maureen knows of many cases through her support group that have been more difficult over a longer period of time than the rather abbreviated, though very traumatic, period that her family underwent with her mom. Mary passed through that terrible stage into a peaceful, content stage. One cannot know what the future will bring. Jim continues to visit three times a week, and even though Mary is mostly nonverbal, she gives him a kiss and rubs his cheek. She occasionally even says "Jim." Whether or not she knows he is her husband will forever remain a mystery, but she knows that he is someone special to her, someone loving and familiar.

Maureen laments the fact that her mother was the last person in the world to whom she would have ever expected this to happen. She worked so hard all her life, helping other people, and had just reached the point where she could finally retire and enjoy life with her husband when struck by Alzheimer's. By the age of sixty-five it had started and at the time of the writing of this chapter, Mary was sixty-eight.

Maureen had called the Alzheimer's Association when all the trouble began. The person she talked to listened to her pour out her story tearfully and then invited her to join a support group. Maureen feels she never would have made it without the benefit of the support group. She remembers vividly someone in the group saying, "In time you will be able to see some of the humor in all of this." She says she went home and told her husband she knew she would never be able to see any humor at all. She now realizes that finding some humor is one of the only antidotes for the intense pain. Love is the most important antidote, of course. But laughter can truly keep us from madness. "Accessing mirth" can help us to heal.

Maureen notes that new members of the support group always react negatively to the laughter at first, as if it is somehow mocking their loved one. With a little time, they usually realize that the laughter is not being directed at the loved one, it is being directed at the cruelty of the shadow side of life.

It was in the support group that Maureen found the only understanding of exactly what she was going through. "No one can possibly understand what it is like to be terrified of your own mother unless he or she has been through something similar. The bizarre behavior is really impossible to understand unless you have experienced it. It feels so good to be told, 'You're not crazy,

I know just what you mean,' or 'I know how to deal with that, I can give you some tips.' It has been such a help."

One cute story that Maureen remembers about her mother involves Jim Palmer, the Orioles baseball player. Mary was always a big fan. Within the past few months, Jim reported that Mary was in the TV room when he arrived one day and had a big smile on her face. He looked at the TV and saw it was Jim Palmer doing a commercial. He chuckled and said, "She doesn't know me from Adam, but she knows Jim Palmer!"

The responses of some of the ladies at the nursing home to Kevin are wonderful. When Maureen and Kevin arrive for a visit approximately once a month, there are three ladies who go through the same ritual every time. The first lady says, "Oh, what a beautiful baby," the second one says, "Is it a boy or a girl?" and the third lady always asks, "What's his name?" Maureen chuckles to think that this ritual may continue even when Kevin becomes a big boy. When she occasionally goes to the home without Kevin, the ritual changes. Then, the first lady says, "Where's the baby?" and the second lady who fusses over Kevin more than anyone says, "What baby?" Maureen responds with, "You know, my baby, Kevin." The lady will then say, "Oh, a young girl like you, you're too young to have a baby!" Maureen really enjoys that comment!

At the present time, Jim is still making his yearly trip to Florida to visit with friends. He was finally convinced that there were enough people visiting Mary and checking on her care. Mary's best childhood friend, who is also a nurse, attends all the care-planning meetings with Jim, to make sure she is getting her fingernails trimmed, hair cut, etc. Maureen says that seeing the friend and Mary together is very touching. She gives her such tender, loving care—the real thing. A treasured friend, who is also Maureen's godmother.

Treasured friends, treasured family, a treasured new grandchild. Alzheimer's is a relentless, devastating disease, but clearly, there can be silver linings here and there.

Postscript

This remarkable family continues to appreciate silver linings—the ones they have experienced in the past and the ones they continue to experience. Kevin is now four and Maureen takes him to visit Mary once a month. (They live at the other end of the state.) He calls Mary, Grandmom Chief. (This is left over from her having been called Chief by her husband when she was supervisor of two floors in the hospital.) Though Mary is verbally unresponsive, when Kevin enters her room, he pulls a chair over to her bed and gives her a kiss. She responds with a smile. When the family is making plans, Kevin always remembers to include Grandmom Chief. Because Kevin has been accustomed to seeing his grandmother this way since he was an infant, he just accepts it. He loves his grandmother and feels loved by her. The family is grateful for that. Jim continues to visit his wife a couple of times a week. He still has the residual effects of his stroke to contend with, but with a good support system of friends and family, he is doing well.

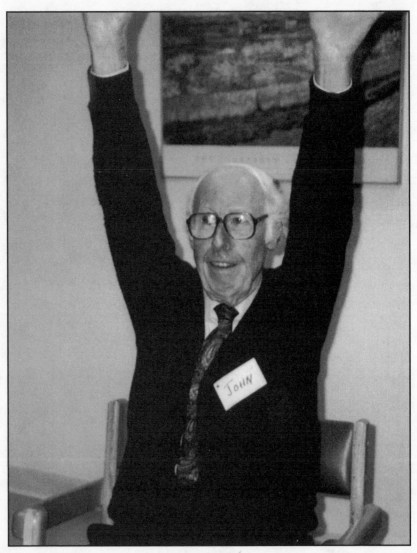

John at Dementia Day Program

Chapter 8

Tales of Temporary Dementia

Not all so-called dementias are true dementias. A neurologist, Dr. Allan Genut, with whom I have worked over the years in the hospital, told me about some of the conditions that can be mistaken for dementia. Fortunately, they are reversible, but needless to say very frightening. All of the following are true stories.

The first case is really bizarre, but its uniqueness makes it a story that should be told. It is about a man in his sixties who worked as a waterman, being out in a boat on the bay daily to catch fish. One day, out of the blue, he tried several times to shoot his wife at point-blank range while she was lying in bed. He missed every time, despite the fact that he was standing right over her. Before placing him in a mental institution, the doctors and police requested a neurological consult. A resident who had worked with this particular neurologist recommended that he examine the man, though he was in a different town.

A year prior to this incident, the waterman had been admitted to a hospital with multiple seizures. He had weakness on his left side, but it was resolved within a week or two of hospitalization and he seemed to be back to normal. If it had been a stroke, he had apparently recovered. It was only after that had happened that he started making these attempts on his wife's life.

During the examination, the doctor asked him why he was attempting to shoot his wife. He said it was because she was having a liaison with an old boyfriend from thirty years ago. The doctor asked him if he had told his wife and her "friend" what he believed. He said he had but that they told him it was a delusion, that no such thing was going on. When asked who this old boyfriend was, he said he was actually a friend of his, that both men had been suitors of the same woman and that he had won. They had remained friends over the years, anyway. He said it was okay to be friends, but he just didn't like this guy fooling around with his wife. The doctor asked him if the other man was at his house at any other time. He claimed his friend, Bill, was with him every day on the boat and that they sat and talked for hours. He admitted that he enjoyed his friend's company, but that he just didn't like the fact that Bill slept in the bed between his wife and him at night.

As is usual in the case of left-sided paralysis, the doctor held up the patient's right hand and asked him whose hand it was. He told the doctor it was his hand. When he held up his left hand and the doctor asked him whose hand it was, he said, "That's Bill's hand." He had actually developed the delusion that the left side of his body, which had been involved in the previous stroke, did not belong to him, but belonged to someone else. He thought that it belonged to Bill. When a CAT scan was done, it turned out that he had suffered a very large stroke in his left parietal region, i.e., in the left hemisphere of the brain. He had denial of his own body parts, which is a syndrome called *autosomatopagnosia*. (Now there's a word for you!) Moreover, he had not only denied that his own body parts belonged to him, but he had to account for them somehow, so he created the delusion that they belonged to his good friend Bill. For over a year, he had actually sat and talked to his own right arm and leg all those lonely times on the boat. When he went to sleep at night, he would mistake his own body as being his friend sleeping between his wife and him. That was why he missed every time he shot, because he wasn't aiming at his wife, he was aiming for where he thought Bill was lying.

This patient flatly refused to have any further workup. The only solution to the problem that was suggested to his wife by the doctor, was to have her change sides of the bed with him. This way, Bill would be perceived to be on the outside, not between them. The neurologist has not heard anything from or about this patient for many years.

A young woman seen by this same neurologist when he was an intern at the University of Maryland Hospital had been transferred from another hospital's emergency room. The patient showed up with a diagnosis of a nonspecific neurological disorder. She was about thirty years old.

The doctor proceeded to examine her. He held up two fingers and she said she saw two. She had some weakness on one side of her face. But what was most peculiar about her was her affect (emotional response). Between the strange affect and the facial weakness he knew he must be missing something. He examined her again, though very seldom did he do a complete neurological examination on someone twice. She passed every test the second time, again showing a very slight facial weakness. She asked to get a drink of water and when told to go ahead, she got up and walked straight into the first wall she came to. She made a ninety-degree right turn and continued to walk straight ahead into the next wall. Again, she made a ninety-degree turn and walked until she hit the next barrier. She did the same thing every time she hit something. It was almost like seeing someone try to navigate a maze, to which an emergency room layout could likely be compared.

The woman got nowhere near the water fountain. At this

point, the doctor realized that she was totally blind and, as impossible as it may seem, didn't even know it. Not only was she blind, but she fooled the doctor on two neurological examinations. He held up a certain number of fingers and she just guessed that doctors usually hold up two fingers. She said two, both times, and got it right. The doctor realized that his neurological exam was completely inadequate and has never been fooled like that again. The patient was admitted to the ward. The next morning, during rounds, the doctor observed her watching a situation comedy on television. She appeared to be watching it intently, though of course she could not see a thing. The team of doctors had her describe all the action on the show and she could describe it perfectly from the dialogue that was going on. They then turned the sound down and asked her to describe the action. She insisted that they had turned off the television and said she wasn't about to describe any action when the TV wasn't even on. In every way, this woman behaved as a fully sighted person. She walked, talked, hit walls (without seeming to care), and headed off to the bathroom whenever she needed to go without ever ringing for a nurse. She insisted that she could see perfectly well though she hit walls face first. Unfortunately, this patient got much sicker and literally did not survive the hospitalization. Instead of just being blind, she became paralyzed. She had a progressive disorder known as *Schilder's disease*, which is an acute form of multiple sclerosis. In her case, it had struck first in the white matter in the back of the brain where the visual areas are housed. So while the gray matter of her visual area was all-intact, that information was being carried nowhere because it was cut off from the rest of her brain. In other words, she had no way of knowing she couldn't see. There was no feedback of information telling her that she couldn't see. It was a bad outcome since she got progressively worse and died after about two months of hospitalization. This was a case of a disease which can be misconstrued as a dementia, when in fact the patient was not at all demented.

There are two cases of "complicated migraine" that were seen by this neurologist. The first was a case of a twenty-eight-year-old man who was clean-cut and handsome, dressed in a three-piece suit, an up-and-coming attorney in a very good law firm. He was on his way one Thanksgiving eve to pick up his family at the airport when he complained to his wife that he was seeing bright lights sparkling in one of his visual fields. It lasted about twenty to thirty minutes and didn't really bother him enough to stop driving. He did complain, however, of having some trouble with his vision. His wife then noticed that his speech became a "word salad." He was speaking complete jargon. They arrived at the airport and were awaiting the family's arrival when he became very belligerent and started actually tearing up the furniture. He was held down by a number of security guards, placed in an ambulance, and taken to the hospital. He continued to be extremely belligerent and had to be restrained.

The neurologist was called in to see him and found that there was no way in the world he could get near enough to examine him. He was so violent that there was absolutely no way of communicating with him. He remained this way for about three days. From the history given by his wife of a previous episode of what is called a *scintillating scotoma*,* followed by confusion, the doctor was able to figure out that he had a migraine. In about forty-eight hours, when he became alert and talkative, of course he complained of the world's worst headache with a lot of nausea. All of the tests, including a spinal tap, bore out the diagnosis of "complicated migraine," in which case patients sometimes become so upset that they are temporarily and nearly completely demented.

There was a similar case of a woman who had a scintillating scotoma as she was driving to an orthopedic doctor's office for

---

*Flashing lights, lasting about twenty minutes, that represent the aura of a migraine. The migraine can stop there or go on to become a "complicated migraine," with sequential neurological deficits.

an appointment. When she arrived at the office and the nurse took her in to change into her gown, she smacked the nurse's hands and pushed her to the ground. Several security officers appeared and had to hold down this sixty-five-year-old woman who weighed about a hundred and thirty pounds. The neurologist saw her in the emergency room and she was practically unapproachable, being both verbally and physically abusive. But this episode only lasted six to eight hours and the patient has absolutely no recollection of any of it. Also, it had happened to this woman once before. This is proof that people who are otherwise intellectually intact can actually become raving lunatics for anywhere from six hours to a day or two. (Not to worry, however, "complicated migraine," to this level, is rare.)

There is another interesting phenomenon that looks a little bit like dementia that is known as the syndrome of *transient global amnesia*. It is not exactly common, but at least fifty or sixty cases have been recorded. Persons who are struck with this condition see things normally in front of them and behave in what can even seem like a normal way. They may even drive twenty miles through the city and back roads, eventually getting to the right place because they recognize each individual intersection or landmark. But if asked where they have to turn, they would have no idea. They can act in the here and now only, so it tends to look very much like a dementia. For example, they may ask about dead relatives or about a spouse who is out of town, and although they are answered, five minutes later they will ask the same question again, over and over. And yet they function normally.

Interestingly enough, there is usually something that precipitates this syndrome. People can have these episodes occur when they do such things as jumping into a very cold body of water, attending a funeral, engaging in sexual activities or an argument, or even during a physical workout. It can happen at a particularly heightened time of emotion and activity. At least a half dozen cases have been seen of executives being hit with it while at board meetings, which can be times of high anxiety. One episode involved the chairman of the board of directors at a hospital. Another involved a man who worked as a publisher. The publisher actually had two such episodes. Both occurred while he was sawing down a tree in front of his house. The first episode happened as he partially sawed down the tree and then six months later he went to saw more of the tree down and it occurred again.

Yet another strange case involved an internist who lived on a farm and raised lambs. Lambskins are supposedly very malodorous if left to hang in a barn for days prior to tanning; sometimes to the point that no one can stand to be near them. The doctor was having an argument with his brother on the phone, when he slammed it down and walked out of the house. He went to the barn and slung a couple of the lambskins over his shoulder. He then proceeded to get in his car and beckon to his wife to join him. He said he was going to his office. She was not able to get in the car with him due to the odor, so instead, followed him in her car. He drove twenty miles from the farm, brought the skins into his office, and was setting up to see patients. Luckily it was Sunday morning and there were no patients. His wife joined him in his office and he said, "Why am I here?" She told him it was Sunday and she really didn't know. He asked again to be told what day it was and then said again, "Well, why am I here?" He kept asking the same questions over and over, and after about two or three hours, had completely recovered and remembered nothing after hanging up the phone on his brother. During the episode this man was actually functioning at a perfectly normal level.

The episode involving the hospital board chairman was recounted by a family member. She and her husband lived on a farm and had their own gas tank. Their car needed a special kind of gas that was put in with a funnel. It was a complicated procedure. When this particular incident occurred, her husband was out of town. She left the house one morning, drove to the gas tank, filled the car with gas, and then drove back to the house. She went to the door and asked the maid where her husband was. The maid told her where he was and she said, "Oh, fine, well then I'm going to work," which is exactly what she had said the first time she left. Next thing, she was at the gas tank, filling up all over again and there was gas running everywhere since the car had already been filled. She drove back to the house, covered with a fair amount of gasoline, and asked where her husband was, once again. At that point, the maid decided to take her to the emergency room. The doctor that first saw her thought she was having a seizure and put her on medication to control seizures. The neurologist saw her a couple weeks later and differentiated the episode from a seizure, calling it transient global amnesia.

Another patient reported having been doing strenuous exercises and the next thing he knew he was standing in his kitchen over the stove, cooking an egg. He went back and checked his book. He had recorded each of his exercises, taken a shower, and driven home. Sitting in his living room, he asked his wife to direct him to the refrigerator. His wife knew there was something wrong, but took him to the refrigerator. He then asked where the dishes and pots and pans were and she told him. When he emerged from the transient global amnesia episode he was sitting at the table eating eggs. The condition is one that usually lasts anywhere from thirty minutes to six hours, with a maximum of twenty-four hours. The episodes are basically all the same with the patient asking the same questions over and over again. The incidence of it happening more than once is 10 percent. The man who had it happen twice while cutting down the same tree was involved both times in strenuous exercise. But it is unknown why, the second time, it happened in the exact same place.

It is not clear what causes these occurrences. It is obvious that they are not the result of seizures because the EEG (brain-wave test) is always normal. A TIA (*trans ischemic attack* or small stroke) is not the cause, because the episode involves both sides of the brain, whereas a stroke effects only one side of the brain. It is not an alcohol blackout because the victims haven't been drinking. So it is called transient global amnesia and most people are not even aware that it exists. Sometimes it can occur as an aura* to a migraine. It is believed to completely delete one's sense of smell, given the actions of the man with the sheep-skins. His sense of smell was perfectly normal after the episode. (Interestingly enough, memory, sense of smell, and emotions are all tied together in the same place in the brain.)

If this chapter seems to have shades of the stories from Oliver Sacks's book, *The Man Who Mistook His Wife for a Hat*, that is because there are definite similarities. The stories in Dr. Sacks's book are longer and more involved, to the point that the book was made into an off-Broadway play.

I felt it was important to include this chapter because, as we all know, sometimes truth is stranger than fiction and, as with all the stories in this book, these stories are absolutely true. Each and every one of them really happened. Sometimes it's a strange world and a little "mirth" can help.

---

*A warning sensation.

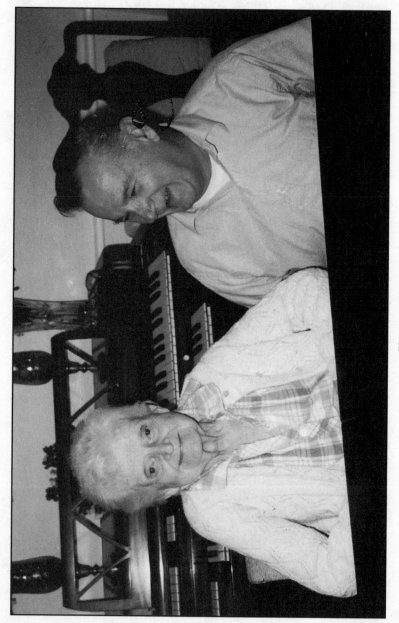

Clara and Tom

Chapter 9

Hospital Happenings

Everyday life in the hospital setting can be very interesting. One becomes accustomed to seeing and hearing just about anything. One of the nurses I know was on the elevator one day when the doors opened to reveal a man standing there stark naked, ready to get on. There were women on the elevator and this event caused quite a stir. One said loudly, "Oh my heavens!" and quickly turned around to face the back of the elevator. My nurse friend took the man's arm and said, "Hi there, come with me, I'll take you back to your room." Fortunately, he obliged. An eighty-seven-year-old Alzheimer's patient, he didn't like wearing a hospital gown and kept taking it and his diaper off. Because his room was not far from the elevator, somehow he had made it there without being seen.

Another funny incident occurred with one of my Alzheimer's patients. She had been sitting up in her chair when I stopped in to see her. I asked her how she was feeling and she said she was doing well. Then she said, "You know, I've been watching all the people going by my door riding bicycles. It is just amazing how

many there are." I was puzzled and wondered if she was halluci-
nating. So I asked her to show me the next time she saw one. We
talked a few minutes and suddenly she pointed and said, "There
goes one now." It was someone going by in a wheelchair! It's
hard to say whether she knew they were wheelchairs and just
couldn't find the word or whether she really thought they were
bicycles. Either way she was being entertained.

One patient was standing with his family in the lounge, looking
out the window. He looked and looked at the view and then
exclaimed, "You know, this looks like Baltimore." His family told
him it was Baltimore. He then turned to a stranger who was sitting
nearby and said, "Did you know you were in Baltimore?"

One of my own most unforgettable hospital stories involves a
patient who had been in the house with her dead sister for
approximately three weeks. When finally discovered, my patient
thought her sister was just sleeping on the floor. She had covered
her with a blanket. Because she was so demented, she had no
sense of the passage of time and probably thought her sister
would get up at any moment. It was also explained that she
would not have noticed the odor because she had gradually
become accustomed to it. This woman had a good disposition,
was generally pleasant, and agreed to go to live in a nursing
home. She basically seemed content with living in the moment
and didn't remember that her sister had died. Mercifully, she had
never been aware of it in the first place.

One of the doctors reported a humorous experience. A female patient of his was in the hospital for a dementia workup. She was able to walk very well and tended to wander. The doctor was sitting at the nurses' station writing in her chart when suddenly a hand loudly banged on the counter in front of him, startling him. It was the patient. She stood tall and erect and said in a loud, haughty voice, "I demand to know who I am and where I have been for the past three years!"

A nurse told me of an incident involving two elderly men in a semi-private room. One was very confused and the other only mildly so. One evening, the more "with it" man stood by his door for a long time without saying anything. Finally the nurses had to tell him to get back into bed. He refused to go and continued standing there. The nurse finally had to go in and investigate. The confused man had had "an accident" and then gotten into the roommate's bed. The roommate couldn't get him out of his bed and he was not about to get into a wet one! Quite good reasoning, actually.

Over the years there have been many incidents that I have experienced but it is difficult to remember them all. One of my patients (we'll call him George) was very confused when hospitalized. He had two daughters, one who lived out of state and one who was a sea captain. We spent weeks trying to find the sea captain who was the one in charge of George. The other daughter said she had been the caregiver for her mother who had recently died. She added that she and her sister had agreed to divide up the parental responsibility and not interfere in any way with the other parent's life. The hospital had to keep this man long past the time when his insurance ran out because the second daughter would not intervene. She just kept telling me to keep trying to reach her sister who was at sea on a yacht. Eventually I reached her through the Coast Guard and Marine operators, but meanwhile, George was getting more and more fractious and had to be kept in a geri-chair at the nurses' station. He had to be watched constantly because he knew how to get out of the chair. He made remarks, many of them not nice, as the nurses went by and he loudly told dirty jokes, usually the same ones over and over. In a way it was hilarious, but after many, many weeks of this it became tiresome. Finally, the daughter arrived and George was placed in a nursing home.

A doctor told me that he had a female Alzheimer's patient in his office one day and was talking to her and her daughter. Out of the blue, the patient reached over and slapped him in the face. The daughter, instead of apologizing or reprimanding her mother, began singing "Row, row, row your boat . . ." With that, the patient began to sing and was distracted. This was the daughter's tool for distracting her mother, and it worked. Meanwhile, the doctor's face hurt!

The family of an Alzheimer's patient, with whom I had worked, discovered a great way to distract their mother when she was agitated. She was at the stage where she liked to tear things up and pick at things or fold papers into tiny pieces. Because of bedsores, they had put heel pads on her at night but she always pulled them off. So they added some masking tape. She still managed to get out of them but did some interesting things with the masking tape, sticking it to her arms or legs. Bath time was always a hassle. They had a bright flash about the masking tape. Before she got in the tub, they took ten small pieces of tape and put them on her knuckles. She intently worked on folding each piece into a tiny square. It kept her busy and distracted during the whole bath. This story is a case in point of being creative with your loved ones, finding ways to distract them from their agitation. It helps everybody involved to stay calmer and feel more in control. *The 36-Hour Day*, by Nancy L. Mace and Peter V. Rabins, M.D., has numerous helpful hints to make life easier for the patient and caregiver.

◆ ◆ ◆

A female patient with Alzheimer's had been becoming progressively confused. She lived with her daughter and family and had been known to say things that sounded strange. She also talked about things that had never happened. One day in the hospital she raised her foot up to show a pink slipper and said, "See these slippers! I have to wear these now, because when I was on the bus the other day, someone got on, came over, and forced me to take off my shoes and ran off with them. And no one stopped him. I can't wait until they pass that crime bill!" Then she added, "And they were my good patent leather shoes." The daughter reassured her she would get her another pair, and next time she came in, she just brought in the pair in question from home, as if they were new.

◆ ◆ ◆

Another co-worker shared an incident with me involving a male patient. This patient's son was concerned about his mother's response to his father's change of mental status. He asked if the social worker would go in and talk to his father. The son felt the father needed to be placed in a nursing home. He constantly insulted his wife and she couldn't seem to understand that he was not responsible for what he was saying, that it was the

Alzheimer's talking. It was causing constant problems. The son also felt that his mother couldn't handle his father's increasing care needs. When the social worker went in the room to see the patient, he was sitting in a chair and greeted her pleasantly. After they talked for a few minutes, the son called her out of the room and told her not to be fooled by his present demeanor. He said that his mother had visited that afternoon. When she greeted her husband with "Hi, Honey," he had jumped up out of the chair, pointed his finger at her, and shouted, "You Jezebel! I know you've been sneaking around on me!" This caused his mother to burst into tears, turn around, and leave. (Believe it or not, these folks were in their nineties.) The son's heart went out to his mother, because a little bit later his father wouldn't remember anything about the incident, but she would still be upset. In the midst of this scene, it would be difficult for the family to glean any humor from it. These are the kinds of happenings that can only be seen as humorous by outsiders, while they also acknowledge the pathos of the situation. Told in support groups, these stories are effective in helping others in similar situations. If a woman were at a support group, brokenhearted because her husband was accusing her of philandering, and she was not able to look at the situation objectively, just hearing a similar story from another wife might relieve her suffering greatly. It could be just what was needed to help her turn things around, take another look, and maybe even be able to "access some mirth."

An incident that occurred in the emergency room was related to both dementia and hearing loss. Which one played the biggest part is anyone's guess. Family members who were waiting with an eighty-five-year-old woman, who was thought to have pneumonia, were trying to cheer her up with any good news they could think of. They told her that her granddaughter had just been appointed director of her department. She said, "What?" They rephrased it: "Mary is now the boss." The grandmother's response was, "She is? I didn't even know she was married."

A psychologist at the hospital told me about her experience with one of my patients, a lady in her late seventies, who had been admitted for change in mental status. She could be heard outside her room talking loudly to herself. When the phone rang at the nurses' station, which was right outside her room, she would call out, "The phone is ringing, is anybody in the bathroom?" After her evaluation, the psychologist told me she had asked the patient where she was and the response was that she was in her kitchen. Attempting to orient her to place, the psychologist explained that she was in a hospital and pointed out the various hospital-type furnishings in the room. She also pointed to the window and said, "Now, that view is not the view you have from your kitchen window, is it?" The woman sat straight up in her bed, looked at her intently, and said, "Young lady, you are not going to fool me. I know I'm in my kitchen. Would you like a cup of coffee?"

Then there is the story of the Houdini acrobat. A lady in her mid-seventies was in a small private room quite a distance from the nurses' station. She was pleasantly confused and it took some people who talked to her a long time to figure that out. She compensated well with her social graces. You could have a fairly normal five-minute conversation with her as long as you didn't ask the standard questions that target onset of dementia. Questions like, "Can you tell me where you are right now, what year it is, what month and day it is, and can you name the president of the United States?" She'd flunk all of those, if anyone were to ask. She was recovering from surgery for a hip fracture when it became clear that she would have to be restrained in her chair or in her bed. She got out of the restraints in the chair and was seen hobbling down the hall. And if this weren't enough, she managed to get out of a double posey (restraints) and climb over the side-rails (there were two on each side and they were fairly high) and somehow get down to the floor. All of this without refracturing her hip—a small miracle! She kept saying, "I just want to go home." Understandable.

◆　◆　◆

A doctor told me about his mother who is eighty-five and lives with him, his wife, and his children. She has been becoming pro-gressively confused over the past two years. He reports that, in her confusion, she seems happy enough. Each morning she begins to sing loudly when she awakens. "Holy, Holy, Holy Lord, God of Hosts" comes the refrain each day. She has gradually transferred quite a bit of what she says to song. If she has to go to the bath-room, which she is very capable of doing on her own, she announces it ahead of time, by singing the praises of the "powder room" and its uses. She sometimes does not remember the names of the other family members except her son, and if sitting alone with him will ask, "Where are the others?" When he asks to whom she refers, she will respond, "You know, the others that live here." Recently, there was a family gathering in their basement club-room—just immediate family. This beloved mother/grandmother, who is still quite capable of navigating steps, came upon the scene and greeted everyone with great excitement, as if she hadn't seen them for a long time. "Well how are you, it's so good to see you, it's been a long time." Everyone was puzzled but accepted the fact that to her it was all new and exciting. They were cheered by her enthusiasm. Another story involved a toothache. She had been complaining about it and her son found her in the bathroom attempting to put roll-on deodorant on her gums. A dentist was the better choice for the cure.

Another doctor's grandmother had a "thing" about her pocket-book. Actually, she had a symbiotic relationship with it. They were "attached at the hip." Everywhere she went, it went, including the bathroom and to bed at night. She slept with it under her pillow. Her obsession was "theft." She was certain someone had robbed her and would accuse anyone she saw of having done so. It was embarrassing when someone outside the family entered the home and Grandma quickly walked up to him and pointed her finger, saying loudly, "He's the one. He stole all my money!" The family finally just had to accept Grandma for herself and let the "mirth factor" enter into the picture. Everyone, in and outside of the family, got used to being accused of theft on a daily basis.

A very nice gentleman was in the hospital for an evaluation for possible Alzheimer's. The nurses were told to keep an eye on him. They were always able to tell when the patient's wife came to visit because the minute she entered the room, he would shout out, "Carolyn, what in the hell are you doing to me now?!" Unfortunately, it reached the point that he thought every nurse who approached him was his wife and shouted out the same thing. Then the staff no longer had the little edge of knowing when his wife was really there.

♦ ♦ ♦

The niece of one of my patients told me not to be fooled by her aunt's seemingly pleasant demeanor. "She has the disposition of a hornet," she warned. Her aunt had stopped speaking to her for two months, at one point, telling her that she was too friendly with her aides. She wanted complete control and felt the niece was giving the aides instructions. "I'm in charge," she said, and banished the niece. Prior to her needing the aides, when she was still living alone in her apartment, she called her niece one day in a frenzy. "Someone has stolen everything from my apartment, the furniture, everything. There is nothing left!" The niece rushed over to find that her aunt had entered the apartment next to hers in error, an apartment that had recently been vacated. When she arrived her aunt bellowed, "They didn't even leave the toilet paper!"

A patient who was in the hospital after having a stroke, told the doctor that even before the stroke occurred, she had been having trouble putting her foot in her mouth. Of course she meant "food" and this word replacement was not resulting from dementia but from aphasia, which is the loss of ability to use words. Hers was very mild, however, and when she realized what she had said, having a good sense of humor, she laughed.

A geriatric specialist, Dr. Michael Gloth, was asking a patient some of the questions needed to establish whether or not he was competent. When he got to the date, the man said it was May 3. The doctor responded that he was close, but that it was actually the fourth. The medical student who accompanied the doctor quietly interjected that it was actually the fifth of May. Touché!

Dr. Gloth also reported that a patient who was demented and in the hospital for a workup, told the staff that he was from Mars.

They all laughed and said, "Sure, whatever you say." Dr. Gloth asked one of the nurses if she was also from Mars, and she responded with, "Not that I know of." They all thought it was just part of the dementia, when it turned out that the patient was, in fact, from a town named Mars in Pennsylvania. The laugh was on them!

In another case, a Hispanic woman told the staff she was the president's nanny and had been for many years. She described how she had taken care of his children. The staff thought this was part of the ruminations of dementia. They were later informed that the woman truly had been the president's nanny, but that it had been the president of Chile and it had been many years ago.

Working in a hospital, one has to find ways to "access some mirth" or one would be overwhelmed by all the suffering. These happenings, though clearly recognized as poignant, help to lighten the load of the caregivers within a hospital setting.

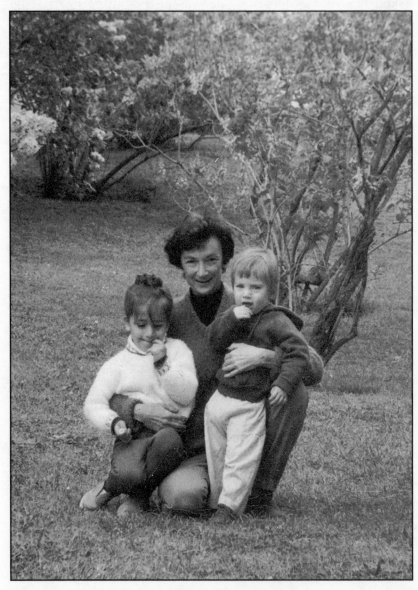

From left: Diane, Gwen, and Robin

Chapter 10

Grandchildren, Nieces, Nephews, and Robin

How do kids fare in all this? What is the role of grandchildren, nieces, and nephews when it comes to giving care to the Alzheimer's patient? It is a very important topic to explore because, as often as not, kids feel like they are second-class citizens and are not considered on the same level as adults. The grandchildren are losing their beloved grandparents, day by day, just as the daughters and sons are losing their parents. The following stories highlight the impact this has on grandchildren, nieces, and nephews and the innovative ways in which some of them handle the situations that arise.

Children are usually very good at maintaining a sense of humor in the face of adversity with the encouragement of their parents. It's a joint effort. So if Mom and Dad seem to be handling things okay, chances are the kids will, too. When Grandma or Grandpa live in the home with the children, there is daily contact. It can become wearing to have the same things said over and over and the same bizarre behaviors occurring again and again.

159

One teenage girl reported that every morning before she went to school she helped her mother dress Grandma, but that before she left the house, Grandma would have undressed at least twice. She felt she had to disrobe completely every time she went to the bathroom. No one could persuade her otherwise. So the family kept their humor intact and just called her "the striptease artist."

As in every other instance, the main ingredient needed here is love. Nothing can be accomplished without it. As the personality of the loved one disappears into the tangles of nerve fibers and the death of brain cells continues to occur, something is needed to give a boost to the family's morale. Something that will help them to get the "periscope up" to look toward a better day. Kids are geniuses at that, because for them, each new day is filled with unexpected hope and they are likely to be able, within that hope, to "access mirth." They will only feel guilty about laughing at Grandma and Grandpa's antics if they are made to feel that way by their parents. If the parents have hit the right wavelength, the kids will probably be okay.

When a sense of humor is maintained and a regular, simple routine is established, the situation can be made manageable. One breakfast-table story I heard involved a grandparent with Alzheimer's, who consistently got up from the table and took her bowl of cereal to her bedroom. She would then return to the table and await her breakfast. Looking at everyone else's cereal, she claimed that she never got any and asked why was she the "only one being starved here?" They would proceed to give her another bowl and the ritual would repeat itself. She would take three bowls of cereal to her bedroom down the hall every single morning. And believe it or not, every day by lunchtime, she had polished off each of the bowls in the bedroom. It was a classic case of hoarding that was probably triggered by some strange fear that she wouldn't get any more food. Grandma never lost any weight, as you can imagine!

The man in the Support Group II chapter had a good story.

He said his eight-year-old granddaughter gave the family a lesson in awareness, in living for the moment. One year, on her birthday, Grandma was having one of her bad days. The family decided that they wouldn't have a big party because they didn't know what would come out of it and what might come out of her. They felt they made the right decision. About a month later this granddaughter asked, "Did you ever give Grandma her birthday party?" They said, "No, she was very sick that day." The grand-daughter's response was, "Why don't we give it to her today? She won't know it's not her birthday. And she won't remember tomorrow that we did it, but she'll enjoy it today."

One of the other participants of Support Group II told the following story: Her son, whom she described as kind, was really as warm and wonderful with both his grandmothers as anyone could possibly be. His grandmother was there one day when he came home and she said, "Bill, where have you been?" He responded, "Out to the library, Grandmother." His mother heard this and thought, "My, he's so short with his grandmother; what's the matter?" Two minutes later Grandmother asked, "Bill, where have you been?" "Grandmother, I was at the library, I have a report to write for school." That was a little bit better. But she continued to ask the same question and each time she did, he would add something to it. "I was at the library because I have a project on science." The next time it was what the project was and the next time he added the number of books that he had taken out. By the time she had asked him ten times where he had been, he had given her the full answer. His mother said, "Bill, you were so wonderful. At first I thought how short you were with your grandmother and then I figured out what you were doing." He replied, "Well, Mom, I knew she was going to ask me at least ten times where I had been, so I tried to make a game out of it. I added something each time to make the story just a little bit different, so it wouldn't drive everyone crazy."

What a great tip that story provides for caregivers! And what a classic example of the way children and young people can accept illness as a part of life, sometimes more easily than adults do.

Another story about this family involved an afternoon in the kitchen. The grandmother and her youngest grandson were making cookies, with Mom overseeing the venture. It took them the whole afternoon to get one tray ready to go in the oven. The wonderful part was that they had worked on this project together. The boy was delighted and would say, "Grandmother and I are making cookies together." It was like seeing two kids at play.

This was a very loving and supportive family. As a show of concern for their mother, the children would leave Mom's slippers by the door in the evening. Mom would come home from work, tired, and find her slippers there. That gesture really gave her a warm feeling. It was the boys' way of letting her know that they were caring for her as well as for their grandmother.

The important point in all of this for the children and young people is that they are being raised to know that people take care of their loved ones. These stories indicate how caring for loved ones is a part of everyday life. Sometimes children are so appreciative of the caregiving. In this same family, one son was actually able to articulate it: "Mother, you are taking care of my father. My father is so important to me and you are the one taking care of him." This was truly a mature young man.

These are good lessons for children since we are living in times when the transmission of moral values passed from parent to child are sometimes questionable. We think of Alzheimer's as a sad disease and we wish no one had it, but it gives us a great opportunity to pass on to our children some of the legends of the family. For example, the Alzheimer's patient talks about things that happened in the past that the children may never hear about otherwise. Early in the disease, long-term memory can be relatively intact. When everything is going right in the family, there is sometimes a lack of depth in the everyday relationships. Fortunately or unfortunately, the reality of suffering often does bring out the best in us. It provides a tension. We learn to live in the moment, appreciate the little things in life, and learn the truth of the old adage "The best things in life are free."

Though many of us may have heard this before, the following story always brings a chuckle. A family was gathered around the table for a holiday dinner. The Alzheimer's patient was the grandmother who lived in a nursing home. Someone from the family visited every day. One teenage granddaughter came out with, "I saw Grandma yesterday and it is so hard to believe she really has Old Timer's Disease." The others tried not to laugh as they gently corrected her.

A nurse's aide at the nursing home where my mother resides told me about her beloved grandfather and her family's journey with him through Alzheimer's. Grandpa had been very active and sharp. But in his late sixties there were noticeable changes that occurred. The family was in denial that it could ever be Alzheimer's. At first it was the usual memory loss, forgetting to lock the store up at night and calling his children by different names. Excuses were made for him. "He has so many kids, who wouldn't get them mixed up?" There were thirteen children. It made sense. He'd be calling one of his daughters and would go through every name until, with great frustration, he would let out an expletive and say, "You know who you are, come here!" During this initial stage, Grandpa would talk about his childhood as if it were happening now. He would say he was going downtown to meet the gang, or going to play ball, or for a soda. He became fonder than ever of curse words and the problem reached the point that he couldn't say one sentence without two expletives in it. The family would just laugh. One of the nephews can imitate Grandpa exactly, so at gatherings he keeps the family entertained by reenacting Grandpa's antics.

This granddaughter went on to say, that in the beginning, everything Grandpa did was cute. Then things started to get tough, as Grandma didn't know how to handle him and would use confrontational tactics that resulted in his becoming too feisty. Paranoia began to set in. Grandpa would sit by the front door every night with a chair nearby to use as a weapon if anyone tried to enter. He constantly peeked around corners and out windows. Finally, it got so bad that the doctor recommended a nursing home. The first one Grandpa was in was unsatisfactory, but they managed to move him to a better facility. Because it was such a large family, someone would visit every day and make sure he was getting the proper care. The nursing home started medicating Grandpa because they couldn't manage him either. Soon, the family observed the slowing down of everything—all systems just basically stopped. This limbo state went on for a few more years until Grandpa died. As a result of this experience, the granddaughter became interested in working in geriatrics and particularly with Alzheimer's patients. Now an aide in a nursing home, she is in a nursing program and has just completed a research project on Alzheimer's. She says the experience with her grandfather helps her relate to her patients. They are all treated as if they were her grandfather. Indeed, this is one dedicated young woman.

The coordinator of a nearby adult daycare program told me an interesting story. Her grandmother had lived with the family when she was a teenager in a small town in rural Pennsylvania. She had been diagnosed as having multi-infarct (multiple stroke) dementia. Both parents worked, but one of them would often come home at lunchtime to fix Grandmother some lunch. However, on other days, Grandmother would order her lunch from a restaurant in town. The family began to notice that three Styrofoam cups would come with the lunch. Grandmother was ordering three martinis, consuming them, eating her three-course meal, and continuing to function just fine. They all wished they had her metabolism!

Another story involved a granddaughter who would kindly offer to sit with her grandmother so her parents could have some much-needed respite time. Grandmother had some stuffed animals and she would often talk to them as if they were real. This particular evening, she was talking about the cat, how nice it was, and how much she liked it. The granddaughter was used to playing along with her, and she started petting the cat and commenting on how much the cat seemed to be enjoying the attention. Grandmother wasn't about to be taken in and rebuked the granddaughter with, "Don't be silly. It's just a stuffed animal." You never know when playing along with an Alzheimer's patient is going to work favorably or cause consternation!

As this book was unfolding, another interesting story came to my attention. It is the story of Robin and her plight with Alzheimer's. Robin is not a granddaughter, niece, or nephew. She is a daughter. But because her story is so extraordinary I decided to include it in this chapter. She was so young that she could have been a grandchild, when her mother first began to show symptoms of Alzheimer's disease. Robin was only six or seven years old at the time. Her mother, Gwen, was in her early fifties. There was one other child, a daughter, who was two years older than Robin.

Robin, now thirty, was courageous to tell me her story. It is quite an amazing one that necessarily involves pain, yet it also clearly highlights the ability of the human spirit to remember the lighter times, even within adversity. The story covers the span of Gwen's life between her fifties and her death at seventy. Robin was twenty-three when her mother died. The diagnosis had been Alzheimer's.

The progress of the disease was fairly slow for an early-onset patient. From the time Robin was six until she was in fourth or fifth grade, things progressed very slowly. But by the time Robin was in sixth grade, the problem was so advanced that even in pictures one could tell her mother was afflicted. The way she dressed was odd, as was her expression. She had become famous for disrobing. Once, the family was in a rather fancy restaurant when Gwen said she was hot and started to take off her clothes.

There was one outfit that she would wear whenever there was a dressy occasion. She refused to buy a new one, preferring to wear the same one over and over. Daily dressing increasingly became a problem. Gwen would constantly be late because she couldn't decide what to wear or how to put it on. Robin's grandmother, Gwen's mother, lived with the family, which helped to provide stability. She lived into her eighties and, fortunately, did not have Alzheimer's.

At one point, Gwen developed problems driving the car. The right-turn-on-red law became a left-turn-on-red law, as well. She probably figured that it made sense. It was quite problematic and there were some near misses before she stopped driving. During that same year, Gwen would often arrive at a destination and say she had no idea how she got there. In those instances, someone would always follow her home. She could usually navigate her way back because she recognized the landmarks, but she wouldn't be able to tell anyone how she did it. That's the way Alzheimer's often works.

Robin remembers quite a bit about her growing-up years and the different incidents that indicated something was wrong. One time, her mother called her at a friend's house and asked her to come home immediately because she was afraid the house would burn down. When Robin arrived, all the kitchen-stove burners were on. Her mother didn't know how to turn them off. Later she said that a friend had come over and turned them on and then had left.

Another incident occurred at the dinner table when Gwen asked Robin to pass the applesauce. Robin didn't do it because the bowl was closer to where her sister was sitting. When her sister passed the bowl to Gwen, she scooped up a handful of the applesauce and threw it at Robin. Clearly, Gwen's impulse control was shot at that point.

Gwen left notes everywhere as reminders. One day Robin had refused to walk the dog. Her mother wrote a note, "walk dog," in order to remember to tell Robin's father about it. Later, when Dad came home and asked what the note meant, Mom couldn't remember. Robin didn't offer any suggestions, thereby avoiding any chastisement. She was a kid and it was a natural thing to do, but she candidly admits that she still has thoughts about the incident and regrets not having owned up.

When Robin had friends in to visit, her mother would often appear wearing her clothes backwards, or inside out. Once, she had put a blouse on as a pair of pants. It happened so often that it was just expected and there was little note taken. Robin's best friend had parents who were alcoholics and she knew Robin's mother had Alzheimer's disease. They offered each other a lot of support. During the day, the friend's parents functioned, and at night they just drank until they fell asleep. Robin is philosophical and says, "In the evenings we just knew to stay away from them. It was all pretty predictable. But with Mom, you just never knew what you were going to get."

Robin had a boyfriend in sixth grade who walked her home and carried her violin for her. Each time he came to the house, the ritual would be the same. Mom would say, "Who's your friend?" Robin would reply, "This is my friend, Tom. Tom, this is my mom." About a half hour later, "Oh, who's your friend?" "This is my friend, Tom. Tom, this is my mom." Robin was so accustomed to this that she didn't blink an eye. But when she looked over at Tom, the expression on his face told her this wasn't normal.

Even in sixth grade, Robin's personality showed a sense of whimsy. She was able to just go with the flow. Her family members told her she was like her mother in many ways. Gwen was a happy person, having had an almost childlike, bubbly personality. Robin worries that she is like her mother in too many ways and that one of them may mean facing Alzheimer's later in life. But even with the family history, she realizes that her chances are not that much greater than the general population. Everyone is at risk and it can strike with no apparent genetic history.

Robin is introspective and able to do the necessary inner work to deal with the pain of her "growing-up" or earlier years. She has been married, has a six-year-old-son, and runs a child daycare business in her home. She also has enough energy left over to lead a youth group on weekends. Nevertheless, she "sometimes feels alone and like a little girl who just wants her mommy." She experienced her mother in dreams years ago, and since she has discussed her childhood with me, those dreams have returned.

Robin feels that talking about the Alzheimer's and opening up old wounds is just what she has needed at this time in her life. She has been able to turn some of the pain into mirth by looking back. For example, she says, it was just understood that on a regular basis there would be a denture hunt. The family would usually find them in the wastebasket wrapped in toilet tissue. Then there was the "blue eye shadow" routine. Gwen always needed a new one. Whenever they shopped, it meant a stop at the cosmetic counter for more blue eye shadow. Her stockpile grew continually.

Gwen started attending an adult daycare program at around fifty-eight years of age. Unfortunately, someone at the daycare center became the proud owner of Gwen's engagement ring. Having a very generous nature to begin with, she had a flash of supergenerosity and gave her engagement ring away. It was never returned.

There was a period when Gwen spoke repeatedly about the "wonders" of having married her husband. She would say, "Can you believe I caught a guy like that?" "Look at my man, can you believe I married him?" That happened around the time the family began to realize something really must be wrong. Soon after, Gwen was taken for a complete evaluation. Robin said that an aunt had made the statement, "There is something wrong with her brain." Everyone was very taken aback by that statement. They thought it was crass. After all, this was Gwenny, and everyone loved Gwenny. She was a delight! "What do you mean there is something wrong with her brain?" Regardless of all the consternation, unfortunately the aunt was right.

Ironically, Gwen always related better to children than to adults. She was a natural as a kindergarten teacher. At parties she would spend time with the children. There was a child who had Down's syndrome with whom she had a great rapport. Interesting, in view of the fact that Down's syndrome victims, if they live past forty, may develop Alzheimer's.* Was there some cosmic intuition or soul connection going on with Gwen? Whatever it was, there was something there that attracted her. A general, lifelong part of Gwen's personality was a love for children and championing the underdog.

There is no need for too much detail about the final years of Gwen's life as they were spent in a hospital. What we seek are bright and happy moments even in the midst of chaos and sorrow. Life has some hard and even cruel lessons to teach us. None of us was ever promised anything more than the moment. If we can learn life's lessons early and savor the moment, we are rich in a special way.

---

*In Down's syndrome, also known as Trisomy 21, there is an extra chromosome 21. Patients with Down's syndrome who come to autopsy, by their thirties and forties have pathological changes in the brain similar to those of patients with Alzheimer's disease, i.e., plaques and tangles.

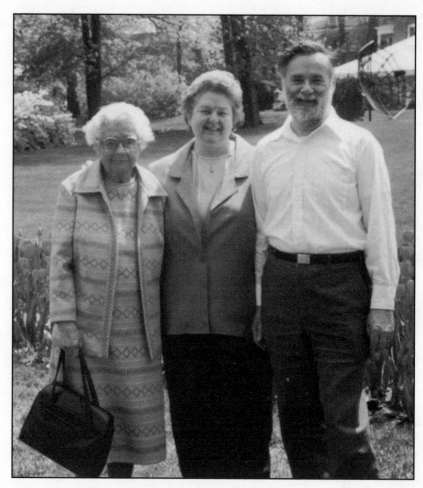

From left: Clara, Dolly, and Tom

Chapter 11

Clara!

You have already met Clara, in the Support Group II chapter. Her star was so high on the "Mirth Chart" that we felt she should have her own chapter. Clara died in January of 1995. This chapter is a tribute to her and to her wonderful family.

Clara had led an active life. She lived alone, had many interests, and loved going places. Widowed for over twenty years and retired for ten, she had marketed in Marrakesh, sampled Spain's sunny beaches, been greeted with a lei in Hawaii, and basked in Bermuda. But then, her life gradually began to fold in around her. Dolly was her only child and they talked on the phone almost every day. Even so, Dolly and her husband, Tom, really didn't know what was happening. There were small signs that went unrecognized at the time. They simply thought she was getting old and old people become forgetful. Her checkbook records were getting sloppy, door-to-door salesmen were having a harvest bonanza, and she couldn't master the new remote control. They tried to get her to have a checkup, but there were always excuses why it would be better later. Alzheimer's was starting its slow, insidious takeover of her mind and life. This was the beginning of Dolly and Tom's years of close contact with the ravages of an illness that was to rule Clara's life. It was also to rule their lives and the lives of their children and children's children for a long time. Through it all, they learned to live with heartbreak and sadness. They also managed to spot some of the absurdities and unexpected twists that come with the job. Humor, in many guises, seemed necessary to survival.

Is It Dark?

Before Clara came to live with Tom and Dolly, they knew things were getting a little strange. One night, at about four in the morning, Dolly got a call from her mother. Clearly, Clara thought she had just taken a little nap and it was afternoon. "Is it dark out where you are? It's dark all over the place here."

Confabulation (The art of creating a full story from partial and poorly recognized facts)

When Clara had first come to stay with them, Dolly and Tom knew something was wrong. Within the first week they were able to get her into the nearby private psychiatric hospital for testing. While Clara was there, some members of the staff told Dolly and Tom that they had been trying to find out about all the excitement they had missed. What they had missed, Clara told them, was a big cops-and-robbers-type fight out on the front lawn, where several police cars and a couple of ambulances were taking care of all the people who had been shot. Apparently, her story was so convincing that even some of the hospital staff members, who knew why she was there, were taken in. It seemed funny that this could happen to people with lots of professional experience. As

Dolly and Tom were confronted with more such tales in the years to follow, it helped to look back and chuckle at Clara's ingenuity.

Confabulation Again

During the interview with the psychiatrist to evaluate the possibility or extent of her dementia, Clara was asked numerous questions about her background. She had always had great respect for doctors and tried to cooperate. He asked about recent events—what she had for lunch, who was president, and also about her husband and other relatives. She failed the lunch and president queries, and continued to regale him with fanciful stories about how one of her brothers had disappeared into the Bermuda triangle, about her husband sailing to the South Pole with Admiral Byrd, and about her other brother who had saved over a hundred people from burning buildings. Dolly and Tom were sitting in the background watching the proceedings. They were amused, as they saw the doctor shaking his head as he made notes. Only after they let him know that those fanciful tales were true did he start looking their way for confirmation or denial of what he was hearing. Most of the things Clara said that seemed believable were from her imagination, while most of the seemingly improbable things were true. Clara had lived an interesting life, surrounded by interesting people.

Stories Change

One of the several times that Clara had fallen and hurt her head, Dolly and Tom had to take her to the emergency room to get her checked out and sewn back together again. As various people asked her what had happened, the stories ranged from falling down the cellar steps to being in the cellar and having six men jump out and beat her up, to slipping while she was trying to help a little girl. There were also several other versions, but none came anywhere near the truth that she had fallen in the dining room and hit her head on the door frame. Every time Tom and Dolly had to take her for treatment they wondered if someone would start to believe her and they would be arrested for abuse or neglect!

Her Teeth

During the years before she came to live with Dolly and Tom, Clara had obtained a full set of dentures. The top ones fit her fairly well, but she never did get comfortable with the lower set. As a result she wore them less and less. By the time she moved in with the family they were no longer in use, and they never saw them. One evening, Clara's grandson dropped over to be with her while Dolly and Tom went out. She suddenly remembered that she didn't know where her lower dentures were. Her grandson searched high and low, to no avail. Finally, when Dolly and Tom came home, their son told them about the lost teeth. They explained that Clara hadn't worn them for years and they didn't know where they might be. Their son had to laugh over the furor that had arisen.

Ready to Go

Sometimes, during the night, Clara would take all her clothes out of the closet and pack them into bags, so that she would be ready to travel when she checked out in the morning. In her younger, healthier life she had done a lot of traveling and perhaps, in her mind, this was just one more of the hotels in which she was staying. Of course, the next morning she would complain that someone had come into her room and messed up all her clothes.

Putting Things Away

Clara's hearing had been bad for years and her family finally managed to get her hearing tested. A hearing aid was called for, but with the Alzheimer's, learning a new skill like putting the hearing aid in or removing it was beyond her ability. Things went fine as long as her daughter handled the daily task. One night, however, she forgot to take it out. The next morning they couldn't locate it. Finally, there it was, sitting in a glass of water, next to Clara's bed. If it's good enough for teeth, why not a hearing aid?

It's a Joke, Son

One afternoon the family was taking one of their many sight-seeing trips, just enjoying the beauty of the countryside. Clara always appreciated such things and it helped make the days go by more easily. Suddenly, Clara exclaimed, "There goes my house!" Confused for a moment, Tom and Dolly spotted the object of her attention. A car license plate had the same number as her street address. The illness was stealing her memory, but the ability to seize the opportunity to crack a joke still lingered.

You Are Only as Old as You Feel

One of the recurring themes for several years after Clara came to live with her family was that she was a teenage girl and had to get to school. Sometimes they told her that the school bus was late. Once, Tom and Dolly decided that if Clara faced reality, she would understand that she was well past the age where she was expected to go to school. Walking with her to the mirror, they had her look at herself. "See, Clara, look at how old you are." "I'm only sixteen. I look older than I really am," came the reasonable explanation. It's useless to try to break through the delusions.

Windows

Before Dolly and Tom resorted to getting multiple locks on their windows, Clara would manage to get hers open occasionally. Once, they caught her climbing out the window, where she would have taken about an eight-foot fall to the ground. However, her favorite use of the windows was in the summertime when they would use the screen for ventilation. That's when her old movie or radio memories must have come back to her, because she yelled, "Help! Murder! Police!" Fortunately, Tom and Dolly never had to talk themselves out of a jail term, since the neighbors understood about her illness.

Dead Bodies

During the first few years, Clara was always seeing disasters occurring around her, usually after she had gone into her bedroom for the night. Often Dolly and Tom would come to answer her calls, to find that she was not alone there. It became a contest between her ability to conjure up dead and injured people and their ability to get them out of her way. For the injured, they could usually get her to accept the story that the ambulance was on the way. Dead people were messier to deal with. Sometimes, they scooped them up and put them in shopping bags. Other times, it was satisfactory to sweep them out of the room.

The Door Keys

It is easy to get lulled into the belief that Alzheimer's patients can't remember. But sometimes they do. One of the ways they managed to keep Clara in the house was to keep the doors locked. As long as she could walk, she never failed to try to open any door she came to, in an effort to get out. One day, she caught Tom at the door and insisted that he let her out. When he told her to use her key, she said that she had lost it. Tom said that he didn't have any keys either. That is when she pointed to the cabinet door where the spare keys were kept and told Tom, "Look in there. That's where they keep the keys."

The Vacuum Cleaner Cover

The family has an upright vacuum cleaner with a cover that is a mama bear carrying a baby bear in her arms (the baby bear is actually tucked into a pouch). Unfortunately, Clara often had a great deal of difficulty interpreting what her eyes were actually seeing and, in her mind, any object could wind up being just about anything else. Usually, things were perceived as living people, which brought up some interesting conversations. One day, Clara was sitting in her chair, with the vacuum cleaner bear standing next to her. She was quite engrossed in conversation with the bear, clearly believing it to be a little girl. The conversation proved to be just a little too one-sided in Clara's opinion, so she started insisting that the "girl" answer her. As she became more insistent, she declared, "If you don't answer me, I'm going to smack your tail!" Not surprisingly, there was still no answer, so Clara lifted up the dress, prepared to give a chastising smack in the usual location, when she stared at the upright post that she found under the dress. Recognizing that what she was viewing wasn't standard anatomy, she dropped the dress and declared with disgust, "You don't even have anything to smack!"

During another episode with the bear cover, Clara and the bear were standing side by side. There was a lot of conversation, which Dolly and Tom heard as one-sided, but Clara may have been hearing the bear answer her. She was obviously enjoying the interlude with the nice "little girl." Finally, as the conversation was drawing to a close, Clara said to the bear, as she leaned over and gave it a kiss, "You're really a pretty little girl, but you sure do have a hairy face!"

At times, Clara and the bear seemed to be hitting it off really well. It was okay when Clara was content to talk to the bear standing near her, but several times she wasn't going to be happy until she got the "little girl" to sit on her lap. First she tilted it over to get it to sit. Then she got it to lie in her lap, but it just wouldn't bend where girls are supposed to bend. Finally, she let the girl stand back up, but it seemed pretty clear to Clara that such an obstinate child had no business with a little baby. So she took the baby bear from her, telling her, "You aren't ready to take care of a baby!"

The Cat

Clara had some stuffed animals that were often real to her. She was happy petting them and she apparently knew that they were animals rather than people, since she never required that they answer her comments. However, Tom and Dolly always had to wash her favorite stuffed cat. It seems that Clara insisted on sharing her ice cream, yogurt, and the like with the cat. When the cat declined to lap up the food, she would hold the cat's mouth down into the treat until she was sure that the pangs of hunger had been satisfied.

Fire

Fire was one of Clara's lifelong terrors. When she went to live with her family, anything that was red or flickering was a fire in her mind. Pilot lights got taped over. They stopped using candles in the house. The fireplace became a mere room decoration rather than a functional part of the living room. After a few years, Dolly and Tom became accustomed to Clara carrying on about it. They found if they just acknowledged her concern, the crisis would usually pass. One day she declared, in a totally unemotional voice, "There's a fire."

"Okay," Tom replied.

After about four more times of emotionless comments, it dawned on them that they were smelling smoke. Either they were moving in with her hallucination or there was more to her story than usual. It turned out that a lamp had fallen over onto the hassock near her and the cushion had begun to smolder. After giving it a glass of water, the situation was well under control. Tom and Dolly had to laugh at themselves this time for being so sure that, with Clara's dementia, they didn't have to pay any attention to any of her emergencies.

Courtesy

One time, when Clara was trying to get out of the house, she was calling to a chair, a broom, or some other object that she perceived as a person. "Please, kind sir, come over here and let me out. Would you please open this door for me?" Then, almost under her breath came the clear, but quiet, "Get over here, you SOB!" Then, resuming her previous sweet tone, she came out with another calm and courteous, "Please, kind sir, I need your help."

Gotcha!

Dolly was washing dishes. Suddenly she realized that Clara had come up behind her with her two hands in the traditional cowboy gunslinger position, saying, "You can't fool me. I know what you're up to." Even though Clara had been with them for seven years by this time, they never could figure out what she must have been thinking.

Don't Confuse Me with the Facts

Clara was constantly striving to get back to her family. In her mind, her mother was sick and needed her. Of course, Dolly and Tom knew what reality was, and in order to help her understand the truth, they had gotten a copy of Clara's mother's death certificate. "That will remove all doubt," they thought. So when she brought up her mother again, they showed her the proof of the error of her ways. "I don't care what that says. I talked to her yesterday, so she can't be dead!" Once again, they learned the folly of attempting to refute "ill logic."

On the Cutting Edge

Clara was watching Tom cut the bottoms out of paper bags to open up to lay out cookies after they were baked. She figured she could make things easier for him. "You don't have to do that," she said. "The other end is already open!"

Daddy's Little Girl

Tom was sitting at his desk, heavily engrossed in some project. Clara went up behind him and began to talk in the voice of a little girl. "Daddy, Daddy, please help me."

Tom was taken aback at the vocal effects and asked her, "Clara, how old are you?"

"Eight," was her reply. Clara had been the apple of her father's eye, and as a little girl, she knew just how to wrap him around her little finger. Old memories stay for a long time, and in her mind, she was back home with Daddy again, using her little-girl wiles.

Makes Sense

Clara was confused. She couldn't figure out why she had to stay in Dolly and Tom's house. Dolly patiently tried to explain that she was sick and this was where she was staying so they could take care of her.

Clara: How long have I been here?
Dolly: Two years.
Clara: What are you doing here?
Dolly: This is my house, I live here.
Clara: How long have you been living here?
Dolly: Twenty years.
Clara: Boy, you must really be sick!

Selective Truth Telling

As time went on, the futility of trying to force concepts of reality onto Clara became apparent to Dolly and Tom. Clara would insist that they tell her where her mother was and so they would reply, "She's over at the park." This seemed to satisfy her. The park they were referring to was Loudon Park Cemetery. Such lies or diversions of the truth are often the only means of satisfying a troubled mind. It certainly seemed kinder than having her relive the grief over the death of her mother several times a week.

Peer Pressure

It was morning. Dolly had set out a pretty dress for Clara to put on for the day, but she was rebelling against wearing it.

Dolly: It's morning, Clara, and you have to get dressed.

Clara: I can't wear that. I have to go to school today.

Dolly: But this is pretty enough to wear to school any day.

Clara: If I go to school wearing that, all the *other* boys will laugh at me.

Clara's memory had been hit by another of the Alzheimer's quirks. This day she was a boy.

Clara's Screen Test

Tom had just added a screen door to the kitchen entrance. Being well aware of Clara's wandering tendencies, Dolly and Tom made sure that the new door had an obscure lock on it, one she wasn't likely to find. It was with a feeling of safety that they left the regular door open and locked the outer door. With the screen insert in place, they figured they would get some of the nice fresh autumn air. For several days, all went well. Clara poked and prodded and felt around the door to find the secret to getting out. But, it was to no avail. Tom felt he had "succeeded." But nothing keeps going well with Alzheimer's. One, too quiet afternoon, they found that Clara had found the key. Her key was a kitchen knife, applied liberally to the screen itself. Once more, they learned that nothing works all the time. It's a game of wits. They found Clara strolling a few blocks away, headed once again for her childhood home.

Summing Up

Tom and Dolly say that there were many events through the years that brought laughter and other emotions, that have slipped from their memories. Some of the laughs were at things Clara had said or done that were so irrational. Others were at themselves and at their stupidity in trying to handle an irrational situation by using logic and reason. Through it all, they felt they had the blessing of dealing with a woman who was basically a pleasant and courteous individual. They also had the support of a caring extended family. It is a shame that through most of her ordeal with them, Clara never knew how much love and support was around her.

Clara lived with Dolly and Tom from mid-1987 until New Year's Day of 1995 when she peacefully passed away. Those years were times of many frustrations for all of them, especially for Clara, but Tom and Dolly both feel that they would try to tackle the situation again, should the need arise. They believe that is what families are for. They are quick to add, however, that there are many situations that would make it impossible to care for a loved one at home and that nursing-home placement is appropriate in those cases. The main thing is to be there for the loved one, showing love and support, whether it is at home or in an institutional setting.

Postscript

It has now been over three years since Clara's death. It took about a year or so for her family to get over the habit of looking into the bedroom or listening for sounds of trouble. Tom and Dolly are getting on with the rest of their lives. Perhaps a few of their own words will provide an insight into this exceptional caregiving family.

"Now it is easier to recall the good times with Clara before she had to deal so courageously with Alzheimer's disease. We are grateful and proud of our children, Claire, Scott, and Tom, who were there whenever we called. Claire, who helped several times a week, was a major instrument in caring for Clara. The grandchildren learned about dealing with the situation at very young ages and were also part of our support system.

"Claire provided frequent respite and company throughout the entire eight years. The last of these respite occasions occurred on New Year's Eve of 1994. Clara had been in a deep sleep for days and was clearly fading. Appropriately enough, the grandmother's clock was chiming away the quarter hours until 1995 made its appearance. (Clara had given us the clock years before.) From about eight o'clock on, with each tolling of the Westminster chimes, Claire told her grandmother how long it was until they could ring in the New Year. Each time, Clara seemed to respond with a slight change in her breathing pattern. At the stroke of midnight, Claire told Clara, 'It's okay now, Grandmom, we saw the New Year in. You can go now.' About five minutes later, Clara took her last breath.

"On reflection, it is clear that during the eight years of caring for her in our home, Clara also helped us. We, our children, and our grandchildren learned more about family, caring, and love. We also learned the importance of being able to laugh at ourselves and at the frequent absurdities of the situation."

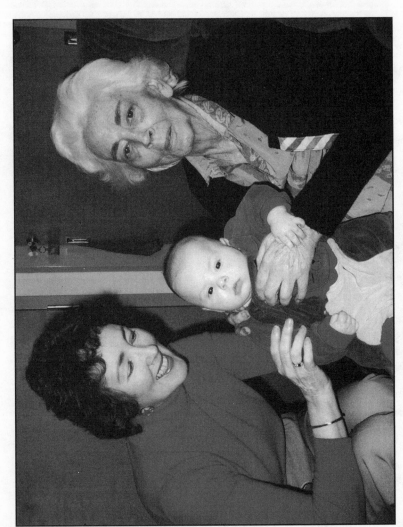

Ellen with Mother and grandson Tommy

Chapter 12

Conversations

I visit my mother nearly every day in the nursing home. During our visits she says the funniest and most amazing things:

When I knew that she would no longer know what the word meant, I showed Mother the picture of Ronald Reagan on the front of *People* magazine in February 1995, with the news that he had been diagnosed with Alzheimer's:

Mother: Oh yes, I remember him.

Ellen: Remember when you asked me why you can't remember anything? Well, you have Alzheimer's disease and so does Ronald Reagan.

Mother: I have? (She paused and looked at the picture.) He has? Well! Nancy will just have to be jealous!

Rolling up a piece of paper into something that looked like a horn and putting it to her mouth.

Mother: Toot! Toot!

Ellen: So, you're tooting your own horn, eh?

Mother: (Looking at me with a wry expression) "You betcha!"

Ellen: (Sneezed)

Mother: Are you getting a sold?

Ellen: What's a "sold"?

Mother: Oh, something you take back to the store if you don't want it.

Ellen: Are you sure you don't mean "cold"?

Mother: (Giggling) Oh well, cold, sold, it's one thing or the other. Sold is like—what's that name—Isolde!

Ellen: You mean *Tristan and Isolde*?

(Gales of laughter follow. Mother thinks these exchanges are very funny. Afterward she is aware that it's a little crazy sounding and will say something like, "It's all gone, there is nothing in my head anymore. Well, I guess it's better to laugh than to cry about it.")

Mother: (Watching TV and seeing something she remembered) Now, once upon a time, I knew something about that, but I just can't remember.

Ellen: Once upon a time wasn't so very long ago, was it?

Mother: It seems more like once upon a century to me!

Ellen: Well, I have to go now, dear. I'll see you tomorrow. (Putting on my coat)

Mother: I like your sweater . . . I mean your tow. Uh-oh (laughing), you know what I was going to say. I like your "towel," instead of "coat." Wouldn't you look cute wearing a towel? I tell you, I just can't be trusted.

Ellen: (At the end of a visit) I'm tired. I think it's time to go home and go to bed.

Mother: We're both in the same box then, because I think it's time that I go home and go to bed, too. (Of course, she meant "boat" and of course, she was home.)

Ellen: Tomorrow is supposed to be a beautiful, warm day. I'm planning to take you outside. We can at least look at the buds on the trees; no leaves yet, but plenty of buds.

Mother: Well, by then I might be alive.

Ellen: It will make me feel alive, too.

Mother: You can't be alive—you're too young.

Ellen: You must mean "dead" then.

Mother: Yes, I wonder what it's like?

Ellen: I wonder, too. Do you think it's a little scary?

Mother: Not really. That's where we're all headed, isn't it? That's what it's all about. After all, God will be there.

When we had been talking about something she couldn't remember.

Mother: Isn't it strange the way things depart your memory?

Ellen: It can happen.

Mother: You can't have everything. But you ought to have something. (Laughing) I can't even talk anymore!

Ellen: Sure you can, you're talking to me now, aren't you?

Mother: Yes, but I think it's best if you do most of the talking because I can hardly remember what I want to say.

While watching TV, a program was lauding the use of certain lingerie. There was talk about "cleavage." Mother started making faces.

Mother: Why does everything have to be sexy? It gets so tiresome!

Ellen: It's just the way society is at this particular point in time, I guess.

Mother: It isn't going to hurt anyone, it's mild enough—but so dull!

Ellen: Would you like me to take you out for a walk in the wheelchair?

Mother: I'll have to "lick" about it. (Realizing she had meant to say "think," she started to chuckle.) I'll do a lot of licking, okay?

Ellen: What did you do today?

Mother: I played golf. You know I've always liked it. (What she meant was she had been watching a golf match on TV.)

Mother: What do you hear about the Great Tonglan?

Ellen: Who?

Mother: I thought you knew.

Ellen: Knew what?

Mother: I lost it—I don't know. (Laughing) Isn't it terrible?

(We have never figured out who the Great Tonglan is!)

Mother: I wish you could stay the night. Can't you ever spend the night?

Ellen: It would be pretty hard, because there is only one bed in here and it's yours.

Mother: Well, you can have my bed and I'll get another.

Ellen: This isn't a hotel, you know, there isn't another room.

Mother: Well, if this isn't a hotel, I'm writing a letter!

Mother: What are you reading?

Ellen: Oh, nothing really, just glancing at this magazine.

Mother: I thought it might be about me. (Laughing) I'm so readable!

Mother: (Saying something that was unintelligible)

Ellen: What was that you said?

Mother: I don't know what I was trying to say. I guess I lost my willpower.

Ellen: How was the group today? (Mother goes to a dementia program daily from 11:30 to 3 P.M.)

Mother: What group? I didn't go anywhere.

Ellen: Yes you did, you go every day.

Mother: You know, I'm a pretty nice girl and all that, but I'm not much when it comes to knowing what's going on. I don't remember being anywhere but in this room all day.

(Mother had only been back from the program for a couple of hours. She has never yet been able to remember that she has gone there. Even triggers, like showing her the nametag that is still on her or a prize she won at bingo, won't jog her memory at this point. It speaks, though, to the contentment she seems to experience by just living in the moment.)

While watching a TV commercial that had a skier going down a hill.

Mother: You know, my friend Ruth and I used to ski when we were about twelve. The first time I skied down the big hill in the back of her house, I fell. But then we skied through the auditorium, where the bodies are buried, and I did fine.

Ellen: Do you mean the cemetery that was near your home?

Mother: I guess. Cemetery, auditorium, why do you have to be so picky?

Ellen: Mother, what's the matter with your eye?

Mother: Nothing that I know of.

Ellen: It looks all red.

Mother: (Grinning) You mean my beauty is being disturbed.

Mother: (Trying to say a sentence that just wouldn't come out) You know, I'm as crazy as a hoot owl.

Ellen: (Laughing) No you're not.

Mother: I wonder who said a hoot owl was crazy in the first place?

Mother: When you're eighty-two you don't know much anymore.

Ellen: Even more years than that have flown by, Mother. You are actually eighty-five now.

Mother: Eighty-five? How do you know?

Ellen: Because I can count the years between when you were born and now.

Mother: How ridiculous, I've been eighty-two all my life and you come along and change it!

While taking Mother for a walk in the wheelchair around the outside of the nursing home, we stopped and spoke to some of the folks. As we moved away from a man and woman we had been talking to:

Mother: I guess that's his wife.

Ellen: What makes you think so?

Mother: Because they live so loosely.

Ellen: I have to go now, I have to attend a meeting.

Mother: Why couldn't you go to the meeting ahead of time, I mean before you came?

Ellen: You can't go to a meeting before it happens, and it's happening now.

Mother: Well, I hope you tell those people what I think of them.

Having great difficulty walking with her walker:

Mother: Merciful Pete! This is hard. (Laughing) Do you think Pete was really merciful?

Ellen: Probably, since someone made up the saying long ago.

Mother: You know, I was in love with a boy named Pete when I was a girl. He lived on the corner of Washington Street in Cumberland.

Mother: (Out of the blue) How does it feel to go to a school without a school?

Ellen: A school without a school, what's that?

Mother: I thought you would know because I thought you went to one. But I'll think about it and let you know.

Mother: I wish Peggy were here to tell you the story from a book—that he got in the car and drove across the wide bar.

Ellen: Drove it where?

Mother: Oh, I wish I hadn't started anything. I'll try to grow it for you later.

While watching swimming and diving on TV:

Mother: I can do that.

Ellen: I know, you were a good swimmer.

Mother: Billy Webber taught me to dive off the switchboard. It was a high one, too.

Mother: (Garbled speech) I'm struggling to say something.

Ellen: That's okay. Don't struggle with it.

Mother: Just put a little common sense in it.

Mother: Getting up from this chair is like coming up from hell.

Ellen: It's good for you though, it keeps your arms strong.

Mother: Dying is probably good for you, too!

Mother had an irritated spot on the side of her nose. We tried putting ointments and bandages on it, but nothing worked. She continues to rub it, the scab comes off, and the whole healing process starts over again.

Ellen: You know you really have to stop rubbing that spot on your nose or it will never heal.

Mother: (Looking at me with great consternation) Why don't you take it home with you and take care of it?

Ellen: It's your nose, Sweetie. It stays on your face and you have to take care of it.
Mother: Oh.

Ellen: Do you remember at all what you did today?
Mother: Nothing at all, except sit around and look at myself.

There was a noise in the hallway that caught Mother's attention.
Mother: What's going on out there?
Ellen: Nothing, it's just someone going by in a wheelchair.
Mother: (Leaning over to look out the door) Get out of my driveway!

Mother: (As I arrived and kissed her) I've been thinking about you.
Ellen: Really? What were you thinking?
Mother: That I love you.
Ellen: (Hugging her) I love you, too.

Postscript

Mother's memory is all but completely gone. Much, if not most, of what she says now is garbled, or unrelated to anything one can understand. She is sharper some days than others and can sometimes say my name clearly. Some things are intelligible all the time. "I love you" is one of them.

Conclusion

> The ultimate lesson all of us have to learn is unconditional
> love, which includes not only others but ourselves as well.
> —Elizabeth Kubler-Ross, *On Death and Dying*

Clearly, this book has been about the search for silver linings for anyone involved with Alzheimer's disease or a related disorder. The old song says there is always one to be found somewhere. It is also about letting in a little fresh air, taking another look, and trying to lighten up. No doubt, it's a tough sell to say that the few lighter moments caregivers can look back on can even begin to make up for their exhausting daily efforts. To the degree that goodness is its own reward, caregivers are rewarded. They know that in their hearts. They are doing a good thing by taking care of their loved ones. And many are confident in the knowledge that if the positions had been reversed, their loved one would have done the same for them. They need to be reminded of that often, because the endless, daily tedium can wipe out any such view of the situation.

The humor presented here has been obtained from real people, from real experiences. All the caregivers and receivers are heroes. In being able to access mirth, they have been able to access the hero within. It is always heroic to face the enemy head on rather than turning and running. Those who are able to keep their sense of humor, while just keeping their senses, as they make this difficult journey with the Alzheimer's-affected loved one have truly made "the heroes journey." They should feel good about themselves and look to the future with hope.

For myself, it has been, to some degree, an exercise in befriending the enemy. Who knows, I may be a victim myself someday. So may any of us, for that matter. But I know, after the years spent on this endeavor, that my life is fuller and richer for the experiences I have had in gathering material for this book. The people I have met and laughed with and cried with, have all been superb human beings—really special people.

So I raise my cup to them and say, "May we all learn to savor the moment, to fully live the life we have to whatever degree possible—be it under advantageous or adverse circumstances."

Suggested Reading

General

Cohen, Donna, and Carl Eisdorfer. *The Loss of Self: A Family Resource for the Care of Alzheimer's Disease and Related Disorders*. New York: New American Library, 1986. Offers practical information on how to recognize serious memory problems, get help, work effectively with Alzheimer's patients, and choose long-term care. Shares personal thoughts and experiences of many persons with Alzheimer's disease and their families.

Coughlan, Patricia Brown. *Facing Alzheimer's: Family Caregivers Speak*. New York: Ballantine Books, 1993. Frank accounts of eight women who cared for their husbands stricken with Alzheimer's disease.

Davis, Robert. *My Journey into Alzheimer's Disease: A Story of Hope*. Wheaton, Ill.: Tyndale House, 1989. A former pastor

197

chronicles his personal spiritual and emotional journey as he experiences memory loss and confusion from Alzheimer's disease.

Dippel, Raye Lynne, and J. Thomas Hutton, eds. *Caring for the Alzheimer Patient: A Practical Guide*. 3d edition. Amherst, N.Y.: Prometheus Books, 1996. Part of the Golden Age Books series.

Greutzner, Howard. *Alzheimer's: The Complete Guide for Families and Loved Ones*. New York: Wiley, 1997. Details symptoms and stages of Alzheimer's disease and reviews what to expect as the illness progresses. Includes tips on coping with behaviors, locating community resources, reducing caregiver stress and family conflict. Addresses possible causes, outlines research progress, and describes physical and chemical changes in the brain.

Hamdy, Ronald C. *Alzheimer's Disease: A Handbook for Caregivers*. St. Louis, Mo.: Mosby, 1998. Covers the presentation, care, complications, and impact of Alzheimer's disease. Also includes the physiological processes of aging and dementia.

Heath, Angela. *Long Distance Caregiving: A Survival Guide for Far Away Caregivers*. San Luis Obispo, Calif.: American Source Books, 1993. Although not Alzheimer's disease specific, this book is one of the few sources that focuses on the problems of long-distance caregiving.

Mace, Nancy L., and Peter V. Rabins, M.D. *The 36-Hour Day: A Family Guide to Caring for Persons with Alzheimer's Disease, Related Dementing Illnesses, and Memory Loss in Later Life*. Baltimore, Md.: Johns Hopkins University Press, 1991. Available from the Alzheimer's Association, 800/272-3900, order no. ED100Z, $9.95; pocket edition order no. ED100ZA, $6.95; Spanish version order no. ED100ZS,

$9.95. Classic, comprehensive guide to home care of those in all stages of progressive dementing illness. Combining practical advice with specific examples, it covers all the medical, legal, financial, and emotional aspects of caring for an impaired relative. Includes chapters on daily care and behavioral issues, medical problems, family relationships, and nursing-home placement.

Manning, Doug. *When Love Gets Tough: The Nursing Home Decision*. Hereford, Tex.: In-Sight Books, 1983. A warm, wonderful booklet that goes step-by-step through the placement process.

McGowin, Diana F. *Living in the Labyrinth: A Personal Journal through the Maze of Alzheimer's Disease*. New York: Dell Publishing, 1994. The author writes of her own experience as a person in the early stages of Alzheimer's.

Pollen, Daniel A. *Hannah's Heirs: The Quest for the Genetic Origins of Alzheimer's Disease*. New York: Oxford University Press, 1993.

Robinson, Anne, Beth Spencer, and Laurie White. *Understanding Difficult Behaviors: Some Practical Suggestions for Coping with Alzheimer's Disease and Related Illnesses*. Ypsilanti, Mich.: Geriatric Education Center of Michigan, 1992. A very practical source of information on coping with Alzheimer's disease. There is a heavy focus on behavior problems.

Rogers, Joseph. *Candle and Darkness: Current Research in Alzheimer's Disease*. Chicago, Ill.: Bonus Books, 1998. Comprehensive report on Alzheimer's research written for the lay public.

Sheridan, Carmel. *Failure-Free Activities for the Alzheimer's Patient: A Guidebook for Caregivers*. San Francisco, Calif.:

Cottage Books, 1987. Describes activities, which can bring moment-to-moment satisfaction to persons with Alzheimer's.

Zabbia, Kim Howes. *Painted Diaries: A Mother and Daughter's Experience through Alzheimer's*. Minneapolis, Minn.: Fairview Press, 1996. The mother, a newspaper reporter, began a diary when diagnosed with Alzheimer's disease. The diary continued until she was no longer able to read and write. The daughter took over with her artwork and some narrative.

Children's Materials

Alzheimer's Association. *Helping Children and Teens Understand Alzheimer's Disease: A Guide for Parents*. Chicago, Ill.: Alzheimer's Association, 1997. Available from the Alzheimer's Association, 800/272-3900, order no. ED209Z; single copies free. Provides parents with ways to help children and teens cope when someone close to them is diagnosed with Alzheimer's disease.

Bahr, Mary. *The Memory Box*. Illustrated by David Cunningham. Morton Grove, Ill.: A. Whitman, 1992. When a grandfather realizes he has Alzheimer's disease, he starts a memory box with his grandson, to keep memories of all the times they have shared. Grades 2–6.

Gold, Susan Dudley. *Alzheimer's Disease*. Parsippany, N.J.: Crestwood House, 1996. Nonfiction presentation of what Alzheimer's disease is and how it affects families. Grades 5–8.

Guthrie, Donna. *Grandpa Doesn't Know It's Me*. Illustrated by Katy Keck Arnsteen. New York: Human Sciences Press, 1986. Available from the Alzheimer's Association, 800/272-

3900, order no. ED103Z, $5.95. A young girl observes her grandfather who has Alzheimer's disease and describes its symptoms and effects. Preschool–Grade 3.

Shawver, Margaret. *What's Wrong with Grandma?: A Family's Experience with Alzheimer's.* Amherst, N.Y.: Prometheus Books, 1996. Youngsters learn that with Alzheimer's there are no simple answers, and that with understanding and love families can embrace their elders and cherish their time together. Grades 2–6.

Spiritual Issues

Cain, Danny, and Bob Russell. *"Blessed are the Caregivers": Practical Advice and Encouragement for Those Providing Care to Others.* Prospect, Ky.: NB Publishing and Marketing, Inc., 1995. Describes caregiving situations and solutions, and gives an inspirational message.

Roche, Lyn. *Coping with Caring: Daily Reflections for Alzheimer Caregivers.* Forest Knolls, Calif.: Elder Books 1996. Each page provides an inspiring daily reflection followed by a related caregiving tip.

Humor

Alzheimer's Association of Greater Washington, 7970-C Old Georgetown Road, Bethesda, MD 20814; 301-652-6446. *Acres of Diamonds: The Importance of Laughter When Nothing Seems Funny.* Bob Grossman, M.S.W., Audiocassette. This tape was made possible by contributions to the Alzheimer's Association of Greater Washington in memory of Ina and Herman Pitt. A wonderful sense of humor and the ability to see "acres of diamonds" allowed them to get through the difficult times.

Cousins, Norman. *Anatomy of an Illness as Perceived by the Patient*. New York: Norton, 1995.

————. *Healing Heart*. New York: Avon, 1984.

————. *Head First*. Viking Penguin, 1990.

Sacks, Oliver. *The Man Who Mistook His Wife for a Hat*. New York: Simon and Schuster, 1985.

Siegel, Bernie. *Love, Medicine and Miracles: Lessons Learned About Self-Healing from a Surgeon's Experience with Exceptional Patients*. New York: Harper and Row, 1986.

Vass, Susan. *Laughing Your Way to Good Health*. N.p.: H. M. R. Publications Group, Inc., 1989. Out of print—can be ordered.

Wooten, Patty. *Compassionate Laughter: Jest for Your Health*! N.p.:Commune-Key, 1996.

Appendix A

Helpful Videocassettes and Kits

A Geriatrics Network. Mental Stimulation For Enhancing Elderly Alertness Kits. The cognitive stimulation created by these kits is wonderful! Deidad Benincasa, 1-800-394-9708. Fax: 561-231-7879. E-mail: **Kits@ageriatrics.com**. Web site: **www.ageriatrics.com**.

Alzheimer's Association. Caregiver Kit. Chicago, Ill.: Alzheimer's Association, 1990. Available from the Alzheimer's Association, 800/272-3900, order no. ED248Z, $399. Includes five videotapes (each runs from 14 to 20 minutes), one audiotape, and three print pieces that provide practical help to caregivers. Great for caregiver support groups!

Alzheimer's Association. Just the Facts & More. Chicago, Ill.: Alzheimer's Association, 1992. Available from the Alzheimer's Association, 800/272-3900, order no. ED247Z, $9.00. Contains twenty-five easy-to-read fact sheets on a variety of topics of interest to caregivers of persons with

Alzheimer's. Topics such as bathing, driving, dental care, and vacationing are covered.

Alzheimer's Association. *Residential Care: A Guide for Choosing a New Home*. Chicago, Ill.: Alzheimer's Association, 1998. Available from the Alzheimer's Association, 800/272-3900, order no. PF110Z. Identifies points for families to consider as they plan for long-term residential care for their Alzheimer's/dementia patient.

Alzheimer's Association. *Residential Care Guide: How to Find What's Right for You*. Chicago, Ill.: Alzheimer's Association, 1995. Available from the Alzheimer's Association, 800/272-3900, order no. PF112Z, $1.75. Describes respite care and the different types for available services.

Alzheimer's Association. *Unidos en la Lucha*. Chicago, Ill.: Alzheimer's Association, 1991. Available from the Alzheimer's Association, 800/272-3900, order no. ED255ZS, $72. Contains two videos (20 minutes and 17 minutes in length) and additional printed material in Spanish in which Hispanic patients and their families share the trials and successes of managing Alzheimer's disease.

Grace. Baltimore, Md.: Video Press, 1991. Videocassette, 58 minutes. Available from the Alzheimer's Association, 800/443-2273. Grace's husband and other caregivers present their practical and emotional solutions to caring for someone with dementia.

Hoffman, Deborah. *Complaints of a Dutiful Daughter*. New York: Women Make Movies, 1994. Videocassette, 44 minutes. Available from Women Make Movies, 212/925-0606. Shows interactions between a person with Alzheimer's disease and her daughter. With humor and love, the daughter discusses how she has dealt with her mother's illness and describes various stages of the disease.

Appendix B

Tips to Reduce Caregiver Stress

The ultimate stress reducer for Alzheimer's will be prevention and cure. Unfortunately, we are not there yet. Meanwhile, the following tips may help:

Early Diagnosis: Recent findings indicate that there are interventions that can enhance the life of a person who is experiencing the kinds of memory loss and cognitive difficulties that may be early signs of a dementing illness. Some dementia symptoms are treatable. See a physician as early as possible.

Educate Yourself: Try to learn as much as possible about Alzheimer's and related dementias. Your local Alzheimer's Association chapter is a good place to start.

Control Stress: Start right away to manage your own stress as well as you can. It isn't easy. Learn to do relaxation exercises, listen to relaxation tapes, get as much physical exercise as possible, and read uplifting material. Religiously plan a time during the day when you can either take a short rest or just "veg out" for a while. This is very difficult if you are the only caregiver—but try.

Community Resources: Your local Alzheimer's Association, Department on Aging, and Department of Social Services can help you find out about the various kinds of support services and resources that are in the community.

Accept Help: Don't try to do it all, it's impossible! Lean on your family and friends a little. They want to help. Try to schedule some time away from your "Alzheimer's-challenged" loved one. Alzheimer's support groups at the Alzheimer's Association, as well as the Helpline, can really keep you from feeling isolated. (Call your local Alzheimer's Association for the Helpline.)

Stay Flexible: Try to stay as open to change as possible, because day-to-day changes in your loved one may surprise or even shock you. The more relaxed and flexible you are, the less likely it will be for your Alzheimer's loved one to have negative reactions.

Legal and Financial Planning: Consult a lawyer who specializes in Elder Law. This is very important. Elder Law is an area of expertise that helps avoid making mistakes in planning. Durable medical power of attorney, living wills, and revocable and irrevocable trusts are important to look into at this time. There are many other key issues also, such as planning for future living situations, i.e., help at home vs. moving to a retirement facility.

Keep Focused on Reality: It is difficult to do, because our natural instinct is to deny this is happening. The progression of Alzheimer's is inevitable until a cure is found. While allowing yourself to go through the natural grieving process for the losses you will feel daily, try hard to focus on some of the more positive moments. There will always be some, obscure though they may be.

Try to Remember: ("that time in September") Remember the song? Keep as many good memories alive and well as possible. Talk to your loved one about happy times gone by. This may reinforce his/her memory. It is so hard to do—but try your very best to smile when you can, and laugh, even when it seems silly. When your loved one sees you smiling, he or she will most likely smile, too. Smiles are contagious! Humor is the best medicine even if you have to "fake it 'til you make it."

Be Guilt-free: Give yourself permission to unload any guilt. There are times when you won't be able to do all of the above. When you are tired and overwhelmed, slow down to a crawl for a while. Take a few minutes for yourself. Put all your guilt into an imaginary balloon and send it out to the cosmos. Give yourself credit—your loved one would if he or she could!

For additional tips and help, call the National Alzheimer's Association Information and Referral Number: 800/272-3900.